LECTURES ON GENERAL PSYCHOLOGY

~ VOLUME ONE ~

LECTURES ON
GENERAL PSYCHOLOGY

~ Volume One ~

DENNIS FORD

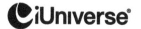

Lectures on General Psychology ~ Volume One

iUniverse books may be ordered through booksellers or by contacting:

iUniverse
1663 Liberty Drive
Bloomington, IN 47403
www.iuniverse.com
1-800-Authors (1-800-288-4677)

ISBN: 978-1-4917-7967-5 (sc)
ISBN: 978-1-5320-0881-8 (hc)
ISBN: 978-1-4917-7968-2 (e)

Library of Congress Control Number: 2015916672

Print information available on the last page.

iUniverse rev. date: 09/30/2016

Also by Dennis Ford

Fiction
Red Star
Landsman
Things Don't Add Up

Humor
Thinking About Everything
Miles of Thoughts

Family History
Genealogical Jaunts
Eight Generations

to twenty five years of students

and to the memory of my Mother,
my first and most important teacher

TABLE OF CONTENTS

PREFACE

In *Thinking About Everything* (entry forty eight) I expressed the insight that our thoughts and experiences will be permanently lost unless we write them down or record them in some way. This insight was a sensible suggestion. It may even have been a sagacious suggestion. And it was a suggestion I did not keep.

For twenty five years I've taught general psychology at the Borough of Manhattan Community College at Chambers St. in Lower Manhattan. That's fifty courses and two thousand students. I came recently to the disturbing realization that there is no permanent record of the twelve lectures I dutifully delivered semester after semester. The only records of the lectures were in the irretrievable notebooks of dispersed students and the cryptic bullet points I outlined on coffee-stained scratch paper. All the good lines delivered in the lectures were in my head—that was a dangerous place for them to be.

I risked losing twenty five years of psychological observations and principles. I couldn't let that happen.

I decided in 2014 to write the lectures word-for-word as I delivered them and then to publish them. This was a way to preserve the lectures and to keep them from sailing to the land of oblivion. The twelve lectures are contained in this volume and in *Volume Two*. The lectures are in the order I presented them. Grammar has been added—speech is sloppy and lacks punctuation—but the content is the same as I delivered in class. Everything I said is now on paper—the material is safe now and preserved. The same definitions. The same examples. The same jokes. The same throw-away lines. The same witticisms. The same insights. The same shrewd observations. The same sage advice. Or so I like to think.

Someone once remarked that teachers are the last vaudevillians. Writing the lectures brought home the truth in that observation. The classroom is my stage. The students are my audience. The blackboard is my set. The chalk is my prop. The lectures are my shtick. After twenty five years I know exactly what works. I know the places in the lectures where I get the students' full attention. I know the places where I lose their attention—this usually happens a half hour before the act ends. I know the places where I shock and surprise the students. I know the places where I bore them. I know the places where they get upset and become earnest. I know the places where they laugh. I know the places where they groan. The groaning doesn't bother me. It's precisely the reaction I expect.

The twelve lectures contain a critical presentation of a selection of mainstream topics in general psychology. For a full exploration of the wonders of psychology the lectures should be read in conjunction with a first course general psychology textbook that covers the same topics. Over the years I used a number of textbooks that are compatible with the volumes of *Lectures on General Psychology*. In former years the textbooks included Bourne and Ekstrand's *Psychology: Its Principles and Meaning*, Lindzey, Hall and Thompson's *Psychology*, and Whittaker's *Introduction to Psychology*. In recent years I favored *Exploring Psychology* by David G. Myers.

Following each lecture I've included a selection of "Tips to Students." These are suggested practices based on psychological principles that, if applied, can facilitate learning the material covered in the lectures. I firmly believe that studying is a skill analogous to throwing a baseball or to surfing. The more students learn the correct methods of study, the better they will get at studying and the greater their performance in class and on quizzes.

I take full responsibility for any errors and for any misjudgments in the applications of psychological principles. As I wrote in *Thinking About Everything* (entry one hundred eighteen), there is no shame in making a mistake. The only shame is having to admit I made one.

OVERVIEW OF THE LECTURES

Lecture One defines psychology as the scientific study of behavior and the mental processes. Reasons for the popularity and the prestige of psychology are explored. The theme of the lecture is the historical and contemporary diversity of psychology. Diversity is examined through the viewpoints of three founders of psychology—Wilhelm Wundt, Sigmund Freud, and John Watson. Diversity is examined through a few of the subfields or specialties of modern psychology. And diversity is examined through the seven perspectives or orientations that provide guidance in conducting and interpreting research. The perspectives are the neuroscience perspective, the behavior genetics perspective, the evolutionary perspective, the behavioral perspective, the cognitive perspective, the psychodynamic perspective, and the social-cultural perspective.

Lecture Two outlines four methods of research used in psychology. The methods are the case study method, survey research, correlation, and experimentation. Examples of each method are given. The contributions toward advancing knowledge provided by each method are examined, as are problems and drawbacks in the use of each method. An overview of science is given. Empiricism is defined as getting data to support theories. Fallibilism is defined as the notion that all theories are incomplete and in need of correction. Students are urged to avoid overconfidence, the false consensus effect, and hindsight bias, and students are encouraged to become educated consumers of research.

Lecture Three describes the vast scope and importance of memory. And it describes the fragility of memory. The memory model is introduced. The processes of encoding, storing, and retrieving are reviewed. The temporal and storage capacities of short-term memory and long-term memory are examined. Long-term semantic, autobiographical, and procedural memories are described. Recognition and recall tests of memory are described. The Method of Loci is offered as a mnemonic. The ubiquity of forgetting is examined in the context of the memory model. The changeability of long-term memory is demonstrated through eyewitness testimony. Factors that contaminate eyewitness testimony, including obtaining post-event information, are specified.

Lecture Four defines learning as a change in behavior due to practice and experience. Classical conditioning is defined as the process in which neutral stimuli acquire meaning. The structure of classical conditioning is described. This structure involves the relationship of the conditioned stimulus – conditioned response to the unconditioned stimulus – unconditioned response. The processes of generalization and discrimination are compared. Operant conditioning is defined as the process in which the immediate consequences of a response influence the rate of the response. The four basic situations or contingencies of operant conditioning are reviewed. These situations are positive reinforcement, negative reinforcement, positive punishment, and negative punishment. The process of extinction is examined in both classical conditioning and operant conditioning.

Lecture Five defines personality as the stable pattern of emotions, motives, and behaviors that characterize a life. Sigmund Freud's theory of psychoanalysis is outlined and evaluated. The concepts of consciousness, preconsciousness, and unconsciousness are described. Freud's tripartite personality theory of id, superego, and ego is presented. The concept of anxiety is introduced, as is the use of defense mechanisms to reduce anxiety. Three trait theories of personality are outlined. The Big Five trait theory of extraversion / introversion, agreeableness, conscientiousness, openness to experience, and emotional stability is reviewed. The trait of internal / external locus of control is described. And the trait of self-efficacy is described with a focus on its importance in interpersonal behavior.

Lecture Six introduces the fantastical marvel of the human brain with a few philosophical speculations. The structure of the neuron is introduced—dendrites, cell bodies, and axons. Events at the synapse involving neurotransmitters are described. The functions of sensory, motor, and association neurons are outlined. The role of myelin and the importance of early experiences in enriched environments are considered as important factors in the growth of the brain and in brain plasticity. The central nervous system and the peripheral nervous system are described. The hemispheres and the lobes of the brain are described in the context of brain localization. Results of the split brain operation are examined. Projection sites for the senses are specified. The role of the frontal lobes in abstract thought is emphasized.

LECTURE ONE ~
The Diversity of Psychology

The journey of twelve lectures and a hundred forty six thousand words sets sail with a definition. *Psychology is the scientific study of behavior and the mental processes.*

If ever there was one, this definition is broad. It extends from the behavior of baseball fans at the Yankee Stadium to what happens when you're alone in bed, asleep and dreaming—but this sounds like a creepy place I prefer to avoid. The definition extends from the behavior of commuters packed in the IND station at 161ˢᵗ St. after the mighty *Yankees* trounced the hapless *Red Sox* nine to nothing to when you're drowsing on the train on the ride home and having a fantasy—but this is another creepy place to avoid.

Psychology is a field that possesses a lot of prestige and power in society—or so psychologists keep telling people. When I tell people I'm a psychologist they become interested in what I have to say. If I don't tell people I'm a psychologist they don't show any interest in what I have to say. Psychology has been one of the most popular undergraduate majors for decades. Psychology is big business. Think of the billions spent in psychotherapy. Think of the billions spent in publishing. If you go into a Barnes & Noble bookstore you'll see a section called "psychology." Next to it is a section of watered-down psychology called "self-improvement." This section use to be called "self-help," but the stores changed the name when they realized customers don't like to think they need "help." "Improvement" is okay, "help" is not okay. (The difference between "improvement" and "help" is the difference between a tune up and an overhaul.) Next to self-improvement is the "parenting and childcare" section. Next to parenting and childcare is a section called "sexuality." In former years middle-aged men in raincoats hung around the sexuality section. In our time yuppie couples in bright clothing stake out the sexuality shelves.

As I say, psychology packs a lot of prestige and power. Psychologists are intimately involved in the education system. Psychologists evaluate students who have trouble learning. They advise whether or not to place children in special education. Psychologists are intimately involved in the business world. Think of the role of psychology in human resources. Psychologists hire, fire, and train people. Think of the art of managing people. Good managers are good psychologists. They get employees to work until they drop. On the way to the floor the employees thank the managers for the opportunities.

Psychology is intimately involved in criminal justice and the legal system. You may not know this, but in divorce cases psychologists play a crucial role in determining which parent gets custody of the children. Psychologists serve as consultants on such issues as eyewitness testimony and the competence of defendants to stand trial.

Obviously, psychology is intimately involved in issues of mental health and clinical practice. Psychologists diagnose disorders and engage in psychotherapy.

Psychology is popular because people are the most complex creation we know of. We are intrinsically motivated to find out who and what we are. We want to know the kind of person he is and the kind of person she is. We want to know what makes him tick and what makes her tick. For that matter, we want to know what makes us tick. From the time our ancestors started walking on two legs we have been curious about what makes people do the things they do. This curiosity started in the Garden of Eden with Adam and Eve asking themselves where they went wrong. Things may have worked out better if there was a family therapist in Eden.

Throughout the history of humanity people have addressed this question—"what does it mean to know ourselves?" The answers to this question are currently phrased in scientific terms. In former years the answers were mostly phrased in religious terms. The answers were also phrased in philosophy and in fiction. Think of all the holy books of the various religions—they are full of psychology. Think of great writers like Shakespeare, Poe, and Twain—their works are full of psychology.

The writers of the great books—the writers of the not-so-great books as well—acted like psychologists in the sense that they observed behavior and commented on the meaning of human existence. Of course, these writers did not see themselves as psychologists.

There is another reason for the popularity of psychology. We live in a stressed-out, nerve-wracking, and dangerous world. Everyone feels anxious. Everyone feels on edge. People need to find comfort and security. People need to find explanations for the bad things that happen—strangely, we're less motivated to find explanations for the good things that happen. We want to know why a person did something bad. We want to avoid similar incidents in the future. We want to find people prone to bad acts before they commit them. Psychology addresses these issues. Psychology provides explanations. Psychology claims it can treat people so disposed. And psychology claims to be able to diagnose these people before they do something vicious or violent. There's a lot of comfort in psychology. That's why people like it and come to it.

Psychology has always been an individual affair, as in the case of the great writers. As an institution—as something we study and attend classes in and get degrees in—psychology began in the late nineteenth century when the people of the time got the idea they could study human beings with the same methods that were used to study rocks and plants and animals. In the nineteenth century psychology gravitated from the individual preoccupation of gifted and thoughtful people to an institution located in universities. We like to think that the people in universities are gifted and thoughtful.

Psychology began with the rise of the now dominant scientific worldview. Psychology contributed significantly to this development. For example, psychology made substantial contributions in methodology and in experimental design. Some people revel in the scientific methods. Other people revolt against them. For the purposes of this course the empiricism that underlies the methods of science simply means that psychologists have to do research and provide evidence for their claims about behavior and the mental processes.

Psychology in America started in a small way. Literally, it involved a small number of men and women—mostly men—most of them known to one another. This was pretty much true until after World War Two when psychology boomed, especially the clinical fields that were founded to help veterans. The professional organization in America is the *American Psychological Association*, commonly abbreviated *APA*. The APA is comparable to the American Medical Association and to the American Bar Association. It publishes books and journals, sponsors conferences and conventions, provides professional training, and addresses insurance issues and financial counseling. The APA is heavily involved with clinical issues. A sister organization, the *American Psychological Society*, focuses on the professional needs of psychologists not involved in the mental health field.

We can observe the growth of psychology in the membership of the APA. When it began in the 1890s, there were a few hundred members. Currently, the membership is well over a hundred thousand.

I've described psychology as a big field—it is a huge field. It is popular, and prestigious, and powerful. I'll like to add another descriptor. This is the word "diverse." Psychology is not a unified field. It never was. There is no "one psychology." There never was. There are a bewildering number of topics and viewpoints within psychology. That's true of our current situation. That's true of psychology's past as well.

What's true of psychology is true of every field of research. Knowledge has grown so exponentially that no person can know everything in a particular field. Think, for example, of physics. There are physicists who study cosmology, which is the study of the origin and destiny of the universe. There are other physicists who study the interior workings of the atom. Quite a different topic than cosmology. Both kinds of researchers call themselves physicists, but they study vastly different topics using vastly different methods.

Think of medicine. When I was a young lad—just a few years ago—I went to one doctor for all my ailments. Maybe you heard of my doctor. He was a kindly gentleman named Marcus Welby. Dr. Welby was called a "general practitioner." He treated anything and everything and he did a fine job. Today, there's no such a thing as a "general practitioner." Nowadays, I go to another physician. His name is Nathan Braunstedder—he's not as widely known as Dr. Welby, although I like to think he does a comparable job. Dr. Braunstedder really doesn't treat anything. If he needs to, he refers me to a specialist—to the heart doctor, to the kidney doctor, to the bone doctor, to the eye doctor, as the case may be. For this referral service, he sends me a bill. I pay the bill through the nose—that's another referral and another specialist.

I'll like to demonstrate the diversity of psychology in three ways. The first way is to compare the views of three of psychology's "founders." The second way is to review some of the "subfields" or "specialties" that exist nowadays. The third way is to review the seven perspectives available in modern psychology.

Wilhelm Wundt (1832-1920) was a prominent German psychologist. We shouldn't hold the fact that he's German against him. Wundt was an influential figure and quite famous in his lifetime, but he's pretty much forgotten today. You'd never hear of him if you didn't take Prof. Ford's general psychology class. Wundt is given credit with founding academic psychology. This took place at the University of Leipzig in 1879—to be precise, it took place on October 22 at 2:30 in the afternoon. I'm joking about the day and hour, but Wundt did found academic psychology. In that year he started to publish research from his laboratory and to call it "psychology" rather than philosophy or biology. Wundt's use of laboratories caught on quickly. By 1900 there were forty two psychology laboratories in the United States, thirteen of them run by his students.

I'll like to mention that I'm an intellectual descendent of Wilhelm Wundt. Angelo Danesino, one of my professors in college, was a student of one of Wundt's students. It may seem I'm dating myself by mentioning this—Wundt died in 1920, after all, but Dr. Danesino was in his sixties at the time and I had him in undergraduate courses in the 1970s.

Wundt believed that psychology should study the *conscious minds of normal people* like you and me—like me, anyway. The method of study was *introspection*, which is the process of thinking about thinking and becoming aware of the thinking process.

Slightly later than Wundt, another and more famous founder of psychology appeared on the scene and offered a different view of what psychology should study. This was Sigmund Freud (1856-1939), who resided most of his life in Vienna, Austria. We shouldn't hold this against him. Freud developed the theory and therapy called *psychoanalysis*. In the lecture on personality I'll outline psychoanalysis, which is fading rapidly in our time and disappearing from the textbooks despite its great influence in America in the twentieth century.

At this time what concerns us is not the theory of psychoanalysis but the theme of diversity. Contrary to Wundt, Freud believed that psychology should study the *unconscious minds of abnormal people* like the people in the room across the hall. The method of research was *dream interpretation.*

Note the diversity. Wundt wanted to study the conscious minds of normal people through introspection. Freud wanted to study the unconscious minds of abnormal people through dream interpretation. When it comes to diversity, we pay our fare and we take our ride.

Slightly later than Freud, a third founder of psychology appeared on the scene and offered a different view of what psychology should study. This was John Watson (1878-1958), who was born in South Carolina, a fact we shouldn't hold against him. Watson was one of the leaders of the movement called *behaviorism*, which was an enormously influential development in American psychology, especially in the area of learning. Many prominent learning psychologists were behaviorists, including B.F. Skinner, whose work we examine in the lecture on learning.

Contrary to Wundt and to Freud, Watson believed that psychology was not the study of the mind, whether conscious or unconscious. Instead, Watson believed psychology should study *observable behavior*. This was the guiding idea of behaviorism—we should restrict our focus to what we can observe. Psychologists should pay no mind to the mind. And psychology should conduct laboratory *experimentation* rather than rely on introspection or dream interpretation as the primary source of data.

It may seem odd that a psychologist rejected the mind as the object of study, but there was logic behind Watson's belief. Watson argued that he could not see the mind. He could only ask, "What's on your mind?" and hope that he get an accurate answer. (If Freud was right, we may not know what's on our mind.) Let me give two examples demonstrating Watson's rationale for rejecting the mind as the object of study in psychology.

When I was a child my mother use to say, "A penny for your thoughts." If she said this today, she'd have to offer me a dollar, maybe five dollars. On one occasion I was deep in dark and unsavory thoughts when she asked. I couldn't tell her what I was thinking, so I lied. I told her I was thinking of the great apple pie she baked at Thanksgiving. "Mom, you make the best apple pie in the whole world." She was so happy when I told her that—I made her day. But I lied. I lied to my own mother. It was for her own good that I lied. She didn't have to know the bad thoughts on her son's mind and, like everyone else, she could use a little positive reinforcement. I hope you see Watson's point. My mother asked what was on my mind and I lied. We can hardly base a science on what could be lies.

Of course, I'm joking with my story about my mother. I never told so much as a single fib to my mother and I never had a thought that wasn't savory. But the theme is serious. We really don't know what a person is thinking. Someone could be staring us in the face and telling us one thing and thinking something completely different. How many times have we watched a news story in which a reporter interviews neighbors of the serial killer who lived in the house next door? What do the neighbors say? "He was such a fine man." "He was a pillar of the community." "I can't believe what they say about him."

I don't ordinarily read *Oprah* magazine, but there was an extraordinary article in an issue a few years back. The article was written by the mother of Dylan Klebold, one of the shooters in the 1999 Columbine High School massacre. He was the goofy-looking blond-haired killer. She describes in tragic detail that Dylan was living a private life of suicidal and, later, homicidal thoughts. She was completely unaware of his death-dealing thoughts. In fact, he wrote journals detailing his suicidal impulses. These journals came to light only after the massacre. He would likely have killed himself if he didn't encounter Eric Harris, the other shooter and a murderous type. Together, they became a deadly pair.

In the article there is a photograph of Dylan three weeks before the massacre. He's sitting at a table. His hair is combed. He wears eyeglasses. He looks perfectly ordinary. He looks perfectly calm and composed. But if we asked him "A penny for your thoughts," we would not have heard the truth. We could never tell from looking at him that he's thinking about murdering his classmates. His mother couldn't tell that. Presumably, she knew him as well as anyone knew him. But she never suspected what was on his mind. Maybe Watson has a point about not basing psychology on what people are thinking. We may hear the truth when we ask or we may not, and we may never know the difference.

We're facing a complex issue at this point. As Watson indicated, we can't base a science on the possibility we may be hearing falsehoods and fabrications. Yet Watson was wrong to ignore cognition altogether. If we wanted to understand what motivated Dylan Klebold we would have to know the murderous thoughts he ruminated over. And if we wanted to learn what was important in his life—what was the most important thing—we most definitely would need to know what was on his mind.

There is another point in the tragedy of the Klebold family. It's a point that is, probably, depressingly common. Many parents do not know what goes on in the lives of their children. Many parents do not know what is on the minds of their children. Busy on their computers and on their cell phones, many children live private lives that are disconnected from their parents and quite at variance from what their parents believe. In the majority of cases this disconnection doesn't lead to difficulties—we trust that there are not many Dylan Klebolds out there concealing malicious hatred. But this disconnection sadly demonstrates the all-too-frequent lack of intimacy among family members. I'm not sure why, but for better or worse, there are parts of ourselves that we conceal from the people we know.

I'll like to demonstrate the diversity of modern psychology in a second way. This is through the use of the *subfields* or *specialties* available in psychology.

The usual course in getting a degree is to go to a four-year college and earn a Bachelor of Arts (B.A.) or a Bachelor of Science (B.S.) degree. Students then advance to graduate school to the master's level (M.A.), which involves an additional thirty six credits of course work and, often, a written research project. The last step is the doctoral level (Ph.D.), which involves an additional thirty six credits and a large scale research project called a "dissertation." Clinical students are required to perform an internship in which they interact with disturbed people under the supervision of an experienced psychotherapist.

Every one of our lectures can be considered a subfield in which students can earn degrees. The American Psychological Association recognizes over fifty divisions or specialties. Some of these divisions include "Military Psychology," "Psychopharmacology and Substance Abuse," "Psychology of Women," "Psychology of Religion," "Exercise and Sport," and "Study of Lesbian, Gay, Bisexual and Transgender Issues." Not to leave men out, there's a division devoted to the "Study of Men and Masculinity."

Let me mention a few prominent subfields. *Experimental psychology*, which is my specialty, is the study of learning, memory, and cognition.

Child psychology is exactly what the name says—the application of psychological concepts to children. *Life span developmental psychology* is the application of psychological concepts across the life span from the cradle to the coffin. This specialty is much in vogue as the American population ages. *School psychology* is the study of intelligence and intelligence testing. Some of you may have had involvement with school psychologists. If your children are doing poorly in school, they will be assessed by school psychologists to check for learning disabilities and the need for special education.

Industrial-Organizational psychology is the application of psychological concepts to the world of business and commerce. We see the application of psychology in consumer issues and in sales. Every successful salesperson is a good psychologist in the sense of influencing consumers to buy what they don't need. And we see the application of psychology in management and in human resources.

An interesting specialty that has grown in importance is *human factors*, which is the study of the interaction of people and machines. Human factors use to be an esoteric field involving the design of space capsules, dashboards, and production lines in factories. It has become especially relevant in our current society in which people incessantly interact with cell phones, computers, and other electronic gadgets. Some people have jobs in which they sit in front of a machine called a "computer" for eight hours a day. These same people go home and sit in front of another computer for an additional eight hours.

Human factors has personal relevance in the sense of making machines user friendly. Human factors also has corporate relevance in maximizing sales. When they first appeared in the marketplace videocassette recorders—remember them?—were programmable only on the machine. This meant that Grandma had to kneel in front of the machine if she wanted to record an episode of *Golden Girls*. This could lead to problems if Grandma left her cane beside the couch. Corporations that progressed to on-screen programming in which Grandma could remain seated and use a remote control device sold more machines and made more profit. Corporations that continued to sell on-machine programming lost sales and went out of business, which is where they belonged for discomforting Grandma.

Clinical psychology is the subfield that studies the causes and the treatments of serious psychological disorders, such as major depression and schizophrenia. *Counseling psychology* is a subfield that focuses on the causes and the treatments of less serious disorders, such as addictions and interpersonal issues like performing better in bed and winning friends and influencing people. The distinction between clinical psychology and counseling psychology is often blurred in the scramble for patients and insurance money, but there is a vast difference between a person who hears voices and a person who wants to give up smoking.

There is a medical specialty called *psychiatry*, which is the study of the causes and the treatments of serious disorders. The objectives may be similar, but there are differences in the training and in the orientation of clinical psychologists and psychiatrists. Clinical psychologists go to graduate school and earn Ph.Ds. Psychiatrists go to medical school and earn M.Ds. Clinical psychologists focus on research and on experimental methodology. Psychiatrists focus on anatomy and on physiology. Clinical psychologists would like to, but in all but a handful of states, they are proscribed from prescribing medication. Like the medical doctors they are, psychiatrists were put on earth to prescribe medicine. The situation with respect to prescribing medication may change in the future as the number of patients increase and the number of psychiatrists dwindle—this would lead to a very different training for clinical psychologists.

This is how it might work for the average person. If you become psychologically disordered, someone may notice that you are acting strangely or saying strange things. If you are employed, this may come to the attention of your manager. You'll be referred to a psychologist who will assess and diagnose you. Diagnosis can be a troublesome topic—we cover this in the last lecture—but it is necessary for insurance reimbursements for medication. If you receive individual or group psychotherapy it will be with a clinical psychologist or with a counseling psychologist. It won't be with a psychiatrist. If you receive medication, a psychiatrist will prescribe it. You'll see the psychiatrist a few times a year to get refills and to be examined. Many psychiatric medications have powerful side effects that need to be monitored and avoided. Most psychiatrists are employed in universities or in private hospitals. There are too few of them to deal with the great unwashed masses of disturbed people.

The histories of clinical psychology and of psychiatry are quite different than what people think. Many people believe that clinical psychology is an old subfield, perhaps beginning with psychology itself. In fact, as a formal subfield in which students can earn degrees, clinical psychology is quite recent. It began after World War Two when the Federal government and the Veterans Administration mandated universities to create training programs in what is now clinical psychology in order to assist veterans who were maimed in the minds on account of their wartime service.

Psychiatry did not always possess the clout it now wields. Until the 1950s psychiatrists were the maintenance men of medicine. No one wanted to be a psychiatrist other than the oddballs who were in need of help themselves—it's always dangerous for patients when the doctors are motivated by personal issues. In the 1950s the first psychiatric medications became available and psychiatry became respectable. Respectability lay in the fact that psychiatrists could write prescriptions. Before the 1950s all psychiatrists could do was scratch their goatees and psychoanalyze people. After that time they could hold their heads high and prescribe meds, something they currently do in great abundance and to little therapeutic success.

I attempted to demonstrate the diversity of psychology through the views of three of our illustrious founders and through the bewildering number of subfields. Let me demonstrate the concept of diversity through what are called *perspectives*.

Perspectives are analogous to worldviews or orientations. Perspectives tell us what kinds of questions we should ask and the kinds of answers we should expect. Perspectives tell us where we should look for information and where we should look for the answers to the questions we phrase. Perspectives tell us what is important in human beings and what we should focus on if we want to study human beings. The perspectives tell us what it means "to know a person" in the scientific sense.

There are seven major perspectives available in modern psychology. They are: the neuroscience perspective; the behavior genetics perspective; the evolutionary perspective; the behavioral perspective; the psychodynamic perspective; the cognitive perspective; and the social-cultural perspective.

The *neuroscience perspective* is prominent today and exceedingly powerful. This perspective says that if we want to study people we need to study their brains. *Brains are us*, this perspective claims. *We are our brains* in ways we are not our lungs or our livers or our sexual organs—I suppose some people are their sexual organs. The study of the human brain, which is an interesting philosophical concept given that the brain is both the object of study and the organ studying itself, has boomed since the 1980s, when it became possible to study the brains of living people in nonintrusive ways and not only the brains of cadavers. We devote the sixth lecture to the neuroscience perspective.

The *behavior genetics perspective* focuses on how genetics underlies behavior and how our personalities result from the interactions of genes and environmental experiences. Like the neuroscience perspective, behavior genetics is a vital and powerful field. I suppose it has been a perspective that has been around since prehistory, given the facts of farming and selective breeding. Its modern version began with the discovery of DNA in the 1950s. This discovery has transformed the world. We do not focus on behavior genetics in this course.

The *evolutionary perspective* focuses on the human species and how our "modern" behavior derives from the history of the human species. This is a controversial perspective and one that overlaps with behavior genetics. We do not cover this perspective in the course, but let me give an example of how the evolutionary perspective may apply to our current situation.

Konrad Lorenz, an ethologist of note in former years, wrote a bestseller called *On Aggression*. (An ethologist is a biologist who studies behavior in natural settings rather than in laboratories.) Lorenz believed that our propensity for killing one another stemmed from our evolutionary history. Lorenz pointed out that animals that can kill quickly, like bears and wolves, exhibit inhibitions or restraints on using "deadly specializations" like claws and fangs on members of their species. There is, of course, violence in nature and animals like bears and wolves kill one another on a regular basis, but in a fight the animal that triumphs usually does not kill the animal that loses and submits. The loser may be relegated to the basement of the pack, but it won't be purposely killed. This is quite different than what happens with humans who blithely kill one another with alarming callousness.

Lorenz suggested that humans lack deadly specializations. We don't have claws or fangs and it's not easy to kill someone with our bare hands. Not that I've tried. Lacking deadly specializations, we never developed inhibitions against killing one another when we acquired weapons such as clubs and bows-and-arrows and handguns and howitzers and mustard gas and napalm and nuclear bombs. Bears and wolves fight tooth-and-nail, snaring sputum close up and snout to snout. In our time drones fly over Afghani targets and a guy in Honolulu presses a button and another terrorist bites the dust.

The *behavioral perspective* originated in behaviorism and in learning psychology. It focuses on observable behavior—on what people do and say. The major concepts in the behavioral perspective are stimuli, responses, and the factors that connect stimuli and responses. These factors are primarily the immediate consequences of responses. Favorable consequences are entitled "reinforcements." Unfavorable consequences are entitled "punishments." We cover the behavioral approach in the lecture on learning.

The *psychodynamic perspective* originated in Freud's view that we should focus on abnormal behavior. The perspective involves clinical and psychotherapeutic elements and it stresses personality factors and the unconscious mind. We are not masters of our minds, according to this perspective, but very much at the mercy of powerful instinctual forces that commenced when we were children. In this course we broach the psychodynamic perspective in the lecture on personality.

The *cognitive perspective* focuses on how we acquire, retain, and use information. We cover the cognitive perspective in the lecture on memory and in the lecture on psychological disorders. This perspective has become a key component in the treatment of depression with its view that depressed people misinterpret events and engage in self-defeating patterns of negative thoughts.

Finally, the *social-cultural perspective* suggests that if we want to know a person we need to know the person's family, friends, lovers, and neighborhood. We need to know what is going on in history and in popular culture as a person develops. The social-cultural perspective sounds quaint in an era of brain scans and genetic tampering. But this perspective is much underappreciated nowadays. We touch on it in the lecture on social psychology.

We often think our own situation—the world we live in nowadays—is the way things always were. This is not the case. Consider that everything we take for granted did not exist two or three decades ago. There was once a time that students did not walk around the campus holding phones in front of their noses. Phones that take pictures. Phones that play movies and music. Phones that connect to the Internet. There was once a time that music was heard on vinyl platters and books were made of paper. There was once a time when people didn't have hundreds of cable stations. There was once a time when people didn't have computers in their living rooms. For that matter, there was once a time when people didn't have computers they could hold in their laps. And can you believe there was once a time when people didn't use microwave ovens to heat up baby's food?

Consider camcorders. When President Kennedy was assassinated in 1963 a handful of movie cameras filmed that horrible event. If we go to any high school football game today there will be hundreds of camcorders filming. The camcorders are so tiny they can be held in the palm. When I was at Fordham we had a camcorder. It was as large as a suitcase. The battery was in a separate case carried by a weightlifter. The film had to be threaded like a tape recorder—it may be you don't know what a tape recorder is.

Consider political developments across the past quarter century. When I was a child the Cold War was white hot. The Western democracies were in deadly conflict with the godless Communist countries of China and the Soviet Union. There were proxy wars everywhere. America was bogged down in Vietnam. The Soviet Union was bogged down in Afghanistan. The world almost came to an end over the presence of nuclear weapons in Cuba. The situation has changed since those tumultuous years. Today, China makes everything we wear and read and the Russians are our bosom pals. We can visit Moscow without a "tour guide" in attendance. We can gloat if we want as we stroll around Red Square. A hawk like George W. Bush claims he looked into Vladimir Putin's eyes and found a man he can do business with. I think Stalin said the same thing about Hitler.

Consider a last example of the social-cultural perspective. One of the greatest killers known to humanity is the disease tuberculosis. The poet Bunyan called it "captain of the deaths of men." If Bunyan wrote that line today he would have to use the word "people" to avoid charges of sexism. But that's another social-cultural example. Tuberculosis killed thousands of Americans on a yearly basis well into the twentieth century. It still kills a million people a year in the developing worlds in Africa and Asia.

In the 1940s researchers at Rutgers University in the country of New Jersey discovered an antibiotic called streptomycin that was effective against tuberculosis. Patients did not believe that any pill could work against so dread a disease. What is more, physicians did not believe a pill could work. So there was a period of time when an effective treatment was not prescribed. Of course, in that period very few pills worked. Until antibiotics became standard doctors really didn't cure anything. They just administered dope—laudanum—that made people forget their ailments.

Think how far we've come. Pills are advertised on television and in magazines. If we go to a doctor and we don't get a pill, we're disappointed. "Please, give me a pill," we appeal, "any pill and don't let your hand cramp up when writing refills." We have pills to fall asleep, pills to stay awake, pills to start having sex, pills to stop having sex, pills to help us lose weight, pills to help us gain weight, pills for every and any malady. Scientists are even working on a pill that will help us forget traumatic events. I suppose not getting a pill is traumatic.

Let's use the examples of anger and of alcohol addiction to see how the perspectives are utilized and how the kinds of questions they pose vary.

With respect to anger we can ask the following questions. Are there brain sites that regulate the experience of anger (neuroscience perspective)? Are there genes that might predispose a person to anger (behavior genetics perspective)? What evolutionary advantage did anger provide—were angry ancestors more likely to survive and procreate (evolutionary perspective)? Is there a personality type that is prone to anger (psychodynamic perspective)? Does the reinforcement of anger lead to its recurrence (behavioral perspective)? Does anger cause people to misperceive and misinterpret innocuous behaviors as threats (cognitive perspective)? What kind of familial events might cause children to grow up prone to anger (social-cultural perspective)?

With respect to alcohol addiction we can ask the following questions. What are the short-term and the long-term effects of alcohol on the brain (neuroscience perspective)? Is there a genetic predisposition to alcohol addiction (behavior genetics)? Did the consumption of alcohol provide an evolutionary advantage in the lives of our ancestors—were cavemen who were boozers more likely to survive and pass their soused genes on (evolutionary perspective)? Is there a type of personality that is prone to overuse alcohol (psychodynamic perspective)? Do the immediate reinforcements of consuming alcohol lead to its over-consumption (behavioral perspective)? How does alcohol affect short-term and long-term memory (cognitive perspective)? Is there a pattern of home life or life in the community that contributes to the abuse of alcohol (social-cultural perspective)?

Let me offer an aside about alcohol and school. I strongly recommend not using alcohol on the days you come to class. Or on the night before you take a quiz. You won't be able to concentrate. You won't be able to remember what you studied. Your grades will plummet along with your reputation.

There are students who come to class seriously hung over. There are also students who come to school under the influence of alcohol. I remember one such student from a few semesters back. His name was Niko. I won't tell you his family name in the event you know him. He was Greek in nationality and came from a place called Brooklyn. He use to stop by after class and chat and tell me how proud his family was that he was attending college. He was the first member of his family to do so. I think his family would have been more proud if he came to school over the influence rather than under the influence. I always smelled liquor on his breath. He finished with a grade of C. Just think how much higher Niko's grade would have been if he managed to attend class sober.

Every topic in psychology can be studied from each of the perspectives. Each perspective makes a valuable contribution so long as we don't believe one perspective is superior to any of the others. Unfortunately, this often happens as researchers come to specialize in one perspective—it's the old story of blind people touching an elephant at different ends. Human beings are so complex no one of the perspectives can capture us. I doubt all seven combined could capture us—capture me, anyway. Odd as this sounds, each of us is more than our brains and our genes and the advantages great-grandpappy bestowed on us and our unconscious motives and the number of reinforcements we have or have not received and our capacity to retain information and our experiences in the home, school, and neighborhood. There is an *emergent* quality in human life that separates us from animals and from the material world.

I believe that this emergent unpredictability in human existence makes people the most difficult topic in all of science to study. This may be the reason why the social sciences are often confused and in a backward state compared to the natural sciences. If I tell a drop of water "You're H2O" it makes no difference to the drop. If I tell a person that "You're extraverted" or "You're creative" or "You're schizophrenic" it may make a great difference. Atoms do not think or have emotions. Galaxies do not generate creative thoughts or suffer psychological disorders. This makes atoms and galaxies much simpler to study—simpler to conceptualize, in any event.

I'll like to point out that nearly everything I said in this lecture is "*in the book.*" I'm going to repeat this phrase throughout the course, "*It's in the book.*" I use the phrase "*It's in the book*" so frequently I've contracted with my undertaker, Earl F. Bosworth of Hoboken, New Jersey, to have the words carved on my headstone. That should give the genealogists of the future cause to wonder. *It's in the book?* "What book?" they'll ask, thinking it's the deed to the silver mine I bought on the Internet.

I would get down on my knees and beg you to read the book on a daily basis, but I suffer from arthritis and I may not be able to get back up. It's a long way from this classroom to the train station and I'd hate to have the Tribeca yuppies staring at me as I pass. I rather think I'm their peer than for them to look down and wonder, "Why is that man walking on his knees?"

It's great to hold class and include the social element in learning, but the most valuable time you'll spend in this course—in any course—is when you're alone and reading the book and thinking about what you're reading.

We've commenced a great journey. This building is our steamship. This classroom is our stateroom. We're going to put out to sea on an intellectual voyage. How long does it take to circumnavigate the world? How long does it take to circumnavigate the world of general psychology? However long, we're on an epic cruise of twelve lectures and a hundred forty five thousand words. Bring your notebooks and plenty of ball point pens and settle in for the voyage on a lounge chair on the sun deck.

Let's hope the ship is not the *RMS Titanic.*

Thank you.

Tips to Students ~
Falling in Love with the Course

If you want to succeed in this course, you'll need to enter into a relationship with it and fall in love with it.

Relationships take a lot of work. Not everyone can enter into one or stay in one. When you're in a relationship you spend a lot of time with the other person. You think about the other person. You talk to the other person and listen to him or her. You want to be with the other person. You make compromises and surrender a lot of things you'd otherwise perform on your own. You give up chunks of your life in deference to the other person. It's the same with this course. You'll spend a lot of time with it. You'll think about it a lot. You'll talk to it and let the book talk to you. You'll want to be in class more than you want to be anywhere else. You'll make compromises and give up a lot of things you'd like to do but can't—or shouldn't—because you're committed to general psychology. You'll give up chunks of your life in favor of the course and you won't regret a moment.

Don't resist the impulse to fall in love with the course—you know it's impossible to resist. Besides, this is your chance to strike out anew and turn your current significant other into an insignificant other.

LECTURE TWO ~
The Methods of Psychology

Do you have theories about people? About their behavior? About their minds? About their relationships? About the things that make them tick? Or are you like the people in Bay Ridge who don't have theories?

If you have theories, how do you know they are correct—really and truly correct? Right now, the old guys in the Wagon Wheel Tavern on Carr Ave. in Keansburg in the country of New Jersey are telling each other how the world works and how the people in the world work. Right now, there are tables downstairs in the cafeteria crowded with students who are telling one another how people work. Right now, there are people waiting on the subway platforms across your land telling one another what makes people do the things they do—on weekends these people have plenty of time to speculate. My point is that anyone can say anything about anything. Talk is cheap and there's plenty of it. That doesn't mean that any of it is really and truly correct.

In science we are committed to saying things that are true. Anyone can say, "This is how people work." They can stop after the period and leave it at that. They're not scientists, they don't have to do anything else. Scientists have the obligation to find out how people actually work. That's not easy, which is why not everyone becomes scientists. It's easier to say whatever pops into our heads and move onto the next topic.

Scientists are governed by two venerable philosophical principles. These principles are empiricism and fallibilism. *Empiricism* means that scientists *have to provide evidence for their claims about how people work*. We want to move from subjective opinion to objective fact.

This movement depends on evidence. On solid evidence. On reliable evidence. On established evidence. On evidence that is incomplete. On evidence that may be open to correction. On evidence that may be wrong.

Fallibilism is the belief—the certainty—that *our claims about the world are incomplete and subject to correction.* Most of the evidence we collect to support our claims can be criticized and revised. This is a point I'll develop in a little while unless something bad happens.

Science is the attempt to describe and explain the world. In psychology we try to describe and explain the people in the world. Description is no easy task. Explanation is more difficult.

According to the standard view, science is an organized body of knowledge derived by specialized methods. The body of knowledge in psychology is organized around specific theories and methods. *Theories express relationships among observed events.* Sometimes these relationships involve descriptions of events that occur together. Sometimes these relationships involve events that serve as cause and effect—these events affect and change one another. In science cause-and-effect relationships are considered to be explanations.

Methods are procedures that scientists believe will result in producing theories that are really and truly correct. People like theories and often overlook the method that produced the theory. The attitude is, "Don't bother me with the details, cut to the conclusions." This attitude is a major mistake. Theories are only as good as the methods that produced them. If the method is inadequate, the theory will be inadequate. If the method improves, the theory improves. Consider astronomy. Thousands of years ago Greek and Chinese astronomers looked at the night sky with their naked eyes and projected mythological theories into it. Centuries later someone invented the telescope and saw farther out—I think this was Hans Lipperhey, but I'm not sure. Different theories emerged. Centuries after that a team of scientists invented the Hubble telescope. They saw farther out. Better theories emerged. Another team of scientists invented something called an X-ray telescope. They saw still farther out. Better theories emerged. Who knows that in the next few years someone will invent a telescope that can peer so far out into space we will see the beings on the other side of the Big Bang looking in at us.

I'll like to stress that science involves an attitude that many people find surprising. Many people have lost their religious faith. They look to science to provide ultimate and final answers. They're surprised when they learn that science has no ultimate or final answers. They're surprised when they learn that scientific theories are incomplete and in need of correction.

Science involves a critical attitude called fallibilism. This attitude is quite different from the religious attitude. Since Darwin's time religion and science have been in conflict. This conflict is unnecessary and unprofitable. Some scientists want to convert everyone to the church of atheism. Some religious people proclaim the holy books are textbooks of scientific facts—they may be textbooks of psychological insights, but hardly of physics, chemistry, or biology. The conflict between science and religion is based on misguided understandings of the attitudes that underlie these two magnificent traditions.

In religion belief and faith are fundamental. Paul calls faith a belief in the "evidence of things that are not seen" (*Hebrews* 11:3). Jesus says, "Blessed are they who have not seen but have believed" (*John* 20:29). In science criticism and fallibilism are fundamental. There are no holy books in science. If there were, the Savior's quote would read, "Blessed are they who have not believed until they have seen and then doubted everything they saw."

In religion obedience is important. We have to obey the priests and the holy books. The *Book of Revelation* (22:19) says that whoever changes one line of the Bible will have his name removed from the "Book of Life." I don't know what that means, but it sounds like something I don't want to find out. The idea in religion is that nothing—or that very little—can be changed. Science involves constant change as false theories are discarded and halfway true theories are amended. Everything changes in science. There are no end points in science.

In religious revivals we hear the congregation answering "Right! Right!" to a minister's observations. In scientific conventions we hear the crowd answering "Wrong! Wrong!" to a researcher's observations.

A foolish book called *The End of Science* was published in 1997. The author, who was a serious science writer, claimed that everything that was knowable was known and that there was precious little to learn. Maybe there were a few odds and ends to collect, but the big picture was complete. The joke was on the author, since something big became known a year after the book was published that rocked physics to the core. In 1998 it was discovered that the expansion of the universe is accelerating. (It was known since the 1920s that the universe is expanding.) It was subsequently discovered that the rate of acceleration increases the farther out we go into the universe. Something is counteracting the force of gravity. This set physics on its head—maybe I should say it set physics on its behind. I'm sure the answers will become known in the future, but right now physicists are positing all kinds of explanations. Dark matter. Dark energy. No one knows what to think. The point is—this is how science works. Our knowledge is always incomplete and in need of correction. If I bought a physics textbook the day before the discovery about the acceleration of the expansion of the universe was announced, I'd ask for my money back.

Somewhere, we don't know precisely where, our theories will come up short. This is counter-intuitive, but science does not progress from being less right to being more right. Science progresses from being more wrong to being less wrong. No matter how sure we may be, our knowledge is always inadequate.

The genius of science is that it has worked out ways to test and revise itself. This is not true in the Wagon Wheel tavern. This is not true in the cafeteria. This is not true on the subway platforms. The best and truest scientific attitude recognizes that our theories and methods can be improved. Theories are tentative and provisional. They provide a glimpse of how the world might work and of how people might work. It's a glimpse made in the blue light of dusk and not in the hot white glare of noon.

It is important that we become sensitive to the uses and limitations of the methods of research. Very few people do research. Research is expensive and time-consuming and we have to know what we're doing, which leaves most of us out. All of us are *consumers of research*. This is true in the small things and in the large things. What toothpaste best whitens my teeth? What shampoo best softens my hair? What skin cream best smoothes the wrinkles? What pills should we take to cure our diseases? How shall we raise our children? How shall we live our lives?

Presumably, the answers to these questions are based on research. Someone somewhere did a study that other people read and apply.

We trek to the supermarket and select one brand of toothpaste over another brand. We go to the bookstore and select a particular book on child rearing. We visit the clinic and the doctor hands us a blue pill rather than a red pill. Why does the doctor do that? Because research suggests the blue pill works better. But how do we know that for a fact? How does the doctor know that for a fact? How do we know the research is any good? We trust our judgment in the case of toothpaste. We trust our doctor's judgment in the case of blue pills and hope for the best.

All research has limitations. All research is based on assumptions, such as a particular statistical procedure should be used or a particular survey captures a trait of personality. These assumptions may be perfectly applicable. Sometimes they are perfectly inapplicable.

The argument is made that the procedures in research should be based on a consensus among experts—we should go with the best established methods and with the theories held by the majority. Agreeing with experts and sharing in the professional consensus may earn us brownie points, but it can be a foolhardy way to proceed. Strange as this sounds, everyone can be wrong. As fallibilism informs us, everyone who shares a theory—everyone who applies a theory—operates with the same incomplete information.

We should also consider that all research is to some degree a sales pitch. Researchers want people to read their work. Researchers want to make a contribution. Sometimes researchers want to make a buck—this is true in the pharmaceutical world of prescription drugs. Sometimes researchers put a better spin on their results than is warranted. Sometimes they emphasize results that make sense statistically but not practically. We want to think positive thoughts and trust what we read, but we have to be wary and remember that a conclusion is rarely final. One study will shortly be contradicted by another study. That's how it goes in science. And that's good science.

Years ago, there was a clothing store called *Syms*. It was located on Route 17 North in Paramus in the land of New Jersey. They advertised that "An educated consumer is our best customer." What's true in buying slacks is true in buying research. If we know how research is done and if we keep our critical faculties on high alert, we can make better choices when it comes to toothpaste, shampoo, skin cream, child-rearing, and medication.

There are three attitudes that impede the scientific process. These attitudes also impede the study of science. These attitudes are overconfidence, the false consensus effect, and hindsight bias.

Overconfidence is exactly that. We are conceited and stuffed full of our own knowledge. We deny it, but deep down we're all know-it-alls. We are sure we are right. And we are sure the other person is wrong. You know you're like that. As soon as I say you're wrong, you become more certain of your beliefs. It goes without mention, but I'll mention it anyway, that no one will be more wrong than the person who's convinced that he or she can't be wrong. All of us need a lot more modesty when it comes to knowledge.

The *false consensus effect* is the tendency we have to believe that *everyone shares our attitudes and traits*. It's the tendency to believe that everyone shares our knowledge and our values. Religious people believe everyone is religious. Materialists believe that everyone is materialistic. Honest people believe that everyone is honest. Crooks believe everyone's crooked. Mark Twain once said—it could have been the guy who served up knishes at Nathan's on the Boardwalk—that "Everyone is free to their own opinion so long as it's mine." All of us need to be careful not to generalize our beliefs where they don't belong and all of us need to be more respectful of the differences among people.

The *hindsight bias* is the tendency *to use old information to prove our theories correct*. We use what has already happened to demonstrate the accuracy of our theories. In a sense, we predict the past. As the saying goes, our lives are lived forward, but understood retroactively. We move toward the future. We understand the past or think that we do. We have to be careful not to use the past to make ourselves look more knowledgeable than we really are.

Perhaps you had a friend or associate who committed suicide. Often you say, "I knew it, I just knew he was going to kill himself." Maybe you did. But maybe you knew what was going to happen only after it happened.

Consider the attack on the World Trade Center. After it happened, many people said they knew it was going to happen, since terrorists tend to go after the same targets. Maybe these people knew it. But maybe they knew it was going to happen only after it happened. They say, "I knew it all along," but they really didn't.

A theory is a complex statement that formulates relationships among events. Theories are creative acts—creative with the proviso that they intend to say something true and accurate about the world and the people in it. Theories are creative with the additional proviso that they say something true that will most likely be found to be in need of correction.

From complex theories we deduce hypotheses. *A hypothesis is a simple statement that can be tested in research.* Sometimes our hypotheses turn out to be correct. More often than not, they turn out to be incorrect. But that's all right. We learn something in being wrong. A particular hypothesis can be removed from consideration.

We need to remember that tests of hypotheses involve many additional assumptions—for example, that we will use particular statistics and methods of data collection and analysis. And we need to remember that not everything can be tested.

Some research is *pure* or *basic*. Basic research is done for the sake of getting information. We want to create an encyclopedia listing every known variable and relationship—this is what the Mormons do with genealogical research. Some research is *applied*. This is research that sets out to solve specific problems—this is what individuals do when they hunt for their great-grandparents among the genealogical troves.

Often basic research turns into applied research. In the 1980s there were biologists working on obscure entities called retroviruses. They were fine people collecting data and filling in the encyclopedias, but no one knew what they were doing. Suddenly there was a disease called AIDS and these obscure scientists became celebrities. Applied research also turns into basic research. To solve the problem of the nature and the cure of AIDS considerable new information had to be acquired. Gathered to solve a deadly problem, this information flowed into the encyclopedias of general knowledge.

I'm going to outline four methods—four ways of collecting data. These methods are the case study, the survey, correlation, and experimentation. I'll define each method, give an example or two, identify the virtues of each, and define what's problematical of each.

I'll start with the *case study method.* A case study is *the intensive study of one person or one group.* Case studies are not the same as biographies.

Rather, they are treatises based on scientific theories and principles. They often serve to demonstrate those theories and principles.

Perhaps the most famous case studies in psychology were those of Sigmund Freud. In science the name of the case cannot be used, so an alias conceals the person's true identity. I sometimes think Freud became famous because of the aliases he assigned. Dora, Anna O., Little Hans, the Rat Man, the Wolf Man—this is to mention five of many.

I'll use the case of the Wolf Man to describe the case study method. The Wolf Man was a young Russian who came to Freud for help. He was what we would call "neurotic." He was filled with anxieties and personality quirks that brought his life to a halt. He had trouble with the opposite sex, he had trouble holding a job, and he was plenty constipated. Freud psychoanalyzed the Wolf Man and concluded that his experiences as a child predisposed him to a life of psychological misery.

Freud really didn't help the Wolf Man—his name is Serge Pankejeff and he lived 1887-1979. No therapist really helped Serge, who spent much of his long life in therapy. There are many people in your country of New York like the Wolf Man. They're good people, but they have obscure psychological problems that complicate their lives. Psychotherapists acquire fortunes not helping them.

The Wolf Man is interesting because he lived to a great age and was interviewed about Freud. This is one of the rare instances in which we have Freud's conclusions about a patient and the patient's conclusions about Freud. Many years ago Basic Books put all the conclusions together and published a volume called *The Wolf Man*. By the way, Serge was called the Wolf Man because he dreamed of wolves. If he dreamed of buffaloes he would have been called the Buffalo Man. If he dreamed of walruses he would have been called the Walrus Man. If he dreamed of moths he would have been called the Moth Man, but I believe that alias was already taken.

Case studies are valuable because we get to learn a lot about one person. We get to learn the innermost core of a person's experiences and development. That's something we don't ordinarily get in this shallow world of superficialities. There are many homes where the adults don't know what goes on in the lives of their children. There are marriages where the spouses are strangers to one another. It's refreshing to get to learn about a person in detail.

Case studies are valuable because they provide leads that may be observed in the lives of other people. So Freud noted what happened to Serge when he was a child. He might be on the lookout for the same occurrences in the lives of other patients. They didn't work too well, but Freud may have noted what psychotherapeutic practices were applied in the case of the Wolf Man. These practices can be applied to other patients as well, probably with equally dismal success.

Case studies provide ideas and open up avenues of inquiry developed using better methods. The important concept of cognitive dissonance, which we cover in the social psychology lecture, originated in Leon Festinger's case study of a group of religious people who predicted the end of the world.

Often case studies are the only ways to get information. There was a case study in sociology of a Mafia family some years ago. We can hardly create a crime family to study, but we can take what's available and observe wherever we can. There have been case studies about mentally disordered people and about geniuses. We can hardly create mentally disordered people or geniuses, but we can study them when they turn up. We get information where we can find it and in the situations nature offers us. The medical literature is full of case studies of individuals who had particular diseases or treatments. In the 1950s President Kennedy was written up anonymously as a case study for his back troubles.

There are problems and limitations with case studies. By definition there is something special about the case. He or she may be a troubled person or a sick person or a criminal or a genius. We need to be careful in generalizing from the case to the rest of humanity. Troubled people may not be like untroubled people and sick people may not be like well people and criminals may not be like law-abiding citizens and the creators of art may not be like the consumers of art. The case study may be different in kind from the rest of us ordinary folk.

Freud didn't think so. Freud believed that by learning about one person—about the Wolf Man—we learn about everyone. People have criticized this view, but maybe there is an element of truth in it. What is the point of reading literature or watching movies if the characters don't reveal truths about humanity at large?

There are social-cultural concerns about the case study method. We have to understand the case in the milieu in which he or she lived—the milieu may be very different than our own time. The Wolf Man, for example, was a gentleman of the old school. He wore a suit all the time. He never drove a car. He never worked the Internet. He didn't use a cell phone. He stood up when a woman entered a room. He watched his language in the presence of ladies. If a woman boarded a bus and there were no seats available, he would give her his seat. Today, if there's one seat left on a bus and a man and a pregnant woman are going for it, she's going to get bumped out of the running. The Wolf Man was a man of his time and his time is very different from our time.

There is a last concern about the case study method. We have to be careful the theorist is not engaged in a complex demonstration of hindsight bias. It is not appropriate to find a case and then fit the theory on the case and claim that the fit proves the theory. Let's pretend I have a theory to advance and I find a case to study. Let's call the case "Ralph." I pick and chose among the facts of Ralph's life. Maybe I stretch things a little. Maybe I ignore contradictory details. When I'm done and Ralph is all wrapped up in my case I proudly proclaim, "See, my theory is correct because it fits Ralph. Or Ralph fits it." This is just too easy. It really doesn't prove anything beyond my creativity in making my theory fit Ralph. Maybe it proves I just pulled the wool over my eyes. The way these things go, I probably pulled the wool over your eyes as well.

The second method I'll like to describe is the *survey*. The survey goes by other names, including *self-report* and the *questionnaire*. The usual procedure is to distribute a list of questions to a group of people. The questions concern a category of behavior, such as introversion or anxiety in personality psychology or opinions about social issues in social psychology. The answers are in the "true / false" format or in the "yes / no" format. Sometimes the respondents are asked to assign a number as the answer, such as "0" for "never" and "7" for "always."

Surveys are the most common research method in the social sciences. They are also common in politics and in marketing. They are ubiquitous because they are easy to administer. Case studies can go on for years. Experiments can be time-consuming and costly. Surveys are quick and painless. I pass out the survey today, score it tomorrow, write up the results the next day, and publish it by the end of the week. By the end of the following week I'm in Oslo accepting a Nobel Prize.

Possibly the most famous surveys in the social sciences were the sex surveys administered by Alfred Kinsey and his team in the 1940s and

1950s. These surveys found that behind the drapes Americans were a raunchy bunch preoccupied with the bottom half of the body. I suppose the situation has grown worse since Kinsey's time. Now Kinsey was an odd fellow who was heavily involved in the sexual liberation of his time. They made a movie about him—you better send the children to the neighbor's when you watch it. Kinsey was born in Hoboken, New Jersey, and lived there for a few years. When I found this out I wrote the mayor asking if a street could be named for Kinsey. There's a street in Hoboken named for Frank Sinatra. Why not for Alfred Kinsey? I never got a reply. Maybe I should have included a return envelop with postage. Maybe I should have slipped a campaign contribution in the envelop. Maybe Kinsey should have recorded a few pop songs.

Surveys are administered to groups called samples. A *sample* is representative of a larger group called a *population*. The answers provided by the sample are supposed to be predictive of the answers the population would have given if it were studied. The Democratic Party can't ask every voter in New York who they are going to vote for. The Westinghouse Corporation can't ask every consumer in the mall who's going to buy their brand of refrigerator. I can't ask every CUNY student how introverted they are or how anxious they are. We can ask a smaller group about their voting, and their purchasing, and their personality characteristics and apply the conclusions to a larger group.

Samples are carefully drawn so the characteristics of the respondents in the sample—age, gender, race, religion, income, socioeconomic status—are proportional to the characteristics of the population. Care is taken that individuals included in the sample are *randomly selected*. Randomization means that *every person in the target population has an equal chance of being in the sample*. Randomization is important for statistical purposes and to prevent bias. The Democratic Party doesn't want to base their predictions only on the voting habits of the upstate farmers. They want the downstate urbanites to be included. The Westinghouse Corporation doesn't want only the wealthiest people to disclose their purchasing habits. They want people of modest means to be included—poor people buy refrigerators, too. And I don't want to include only the most introverted or the most anxious people in my study. I want a broad range of individuals to take the survey.

Surveys are usually quite modest in their scope and in their goals. This is a strength of survey research. I don't want to know about your childhood and how everyone in grade school picked on you. I just want to know who you'll vote for. I don't want to know how your parents mistreated you. All I want to know is whether you'll buy a Westinghouse refrigerator. And I don't want to know your unsavory fantasies. All I want to know is how introverted you are.

Case study research can be considered a type of vertical research. It drills deep into the case, allowing all the savory and unsavory elements to ooze to the surface. Survey research can be considered a type of horizontal research. It doesn't drill deep into the life stories of the participants. It stays at the surface and accumulates facts about specific topics.

Despite the ease and efficiency of survey research, care must be taken in drawing conclusions based on surveys. Maybe the term is "because of" rather than "despite." We have to be careful consumers when it comes to survey research.

We need to be especially sensitive to the composition of the sample. We need to ask whether there is anything special about the individuals who comprise the sample and whether there may be subtle biases in the sample. Strange as this sounds, it's useful to know who's not included in the sample. And we have to be careful to ascertain whether data from one kind of sample is used to make predictions about a different kind of population.

Perhaps the most famous incident of *sampling error* or *selection bias* occurred in the 1936 presidential election between Franklin Roosevelt and Alfred Landon. The *Literary Digest* was a well-respected magazine that had a track record for predicting who would win presidential elections. Their poll involved a mailing of ten million surveys. (The return was poor—less than three million responses.) Based on these responses the *Digest* predicted that Landon would trounce Roosevelt. In fact, the opposite happened. Roosevelt trounced Landon, handily. The magazine based its mailing on telephone directories and on club and association memberships. They failed to realize that only middle-and-upper class voters had phones in 1936 or belonged to clubs and associations. These people indicated they would vote for the Republican Landon. There were a lot more poor people in 1936 than middle-and-upper class people and the poor voted for the Democrat Roosevelt.

The large number of non-responses indicates an additional issue with surveys. Survey results are based only on the people who answer the surveys. How's that for an obvious statement? There is no way to know how non-responders would answer the survey. There may be differences in the characteristics of people who respond to surveys and those who do not. Our conclusions may be quite different if we could magically discover how the non-responders would have answered the survey.

Consider using one kind of sample to make predictions about a different kind of population. There is likely a vast difference between the shoppers in the Short Hills Mall in New Jersey and the shoppers in the Mall at 34th St. in the old E.J. Korvette building. It would be a mistake—it would cost boxcars of money—if retailers used survey data from the shoppers in the Short Hills Mall to predict what the shoppers in the 34th St. Mall will buy. And the same is true using Midtown New York shoppers to predict the behavior of the shoppers in suburban Short Hills.

There are other problems with survey research. We have to consider the research topic. People may readily and accurately disclose their preferences about clothing and electronic gadgets. People may passionately disclose the names of their favorite candidates for office. And people may be more circumspect about disclosing their sexual practices, their addictions, and their salaries. Questions about how many vegetables we eat in a week will likely produce an honest reply. Questions about how many alcoholic beverages we consume in a week may not. Questions about how many newspapers a week we read will likely be answered more accurately than questions about how many sexual trysts we engaged in.

Or they may not. Even seemingly innocuous topics like vegetable consumption and civics can be open to misrepresentation. Many years ago the creators of surveys became aware of a potent variable that can lead to misleading results. The variable is called *social desirability*, which involves the all-too-human motive of *presenting ourselves in the best possible light*. We always want to look good and to have other people think highly of us. It's embarrassing to admit to boozing and to sexual peccadilloes. After all, we're supposed to have manners and good morals. It's also embarrassing to admit that we do not eat vegetables or read newspapers. After all, we're supposed to eat healthy and to be informed citizens. We may deflate the numbers of drinks and trysts. We may inflate the carrots and broccoli and we may claim we use the New York *Times* as a fly swatter after we complete the crossword puzzle.

There are other issues in survey research. The *wording of questions* may affect the kinds of answers people provide. Are you pro-choice or anti-life? Are you pro-life or anti-choice? There's an apocryphal story about a Catholic nun who smoked. She asked the Mother Superior if she could smoke while she prayed. "Of course, you can't smoke while you pray," Mother Superior informed her with a "tsk" for the asking. The nun reversed the question and asked if she could pray while she smoked. "Of course, you can pray while you smoke," Mother Superior replied with an "arrr" for being bothered.

The wording of questions plays an important role in memory research and in eyewitness testimony, as you'll hear in the next lecture. Elizabeth Loftus was a preeminent experimenter in eyewitness testimony. In one of her experiments she stages a crime while giving a lecture. Someone runs into the classroom and grabs her purse, which lies on the desk. The students in the class have become eyewitnesses to a crime. She hands out questionnaires asking about details of the crime. Was the perp—that's short for perpetrator, something I once heard on an episode of *Law and Order*—wearing jeans or dress slacks? What color was his pants? What color was his shirt? Was his shirt short sleeve or long sleeve? What color was his hair? How was his hair parted? One of the questions is the manipulation of the experiment. Half the students are asked, "How *short* was the perp?" Half the students are asked, "How *tall* was the perp?" Changing one word—short to tall—changes the average estimate of the perp's height by a few inches.

Words are powerful things. Even wee tiny words like "a" and "the" are powerful. Consider this example. You're a witness to a crime, but you're not sure whether the perp had a gun. A police officer runs up and asks, "Did you see *a* gun?" You're not sure and the officer seems not to be sure. You answer truthfully, "No, officer, I don't think I saw a gun." Change the scenario by one word. The police officer now asks, "Did you see *the* gun?" You're not sure—you're not unsure either. The officer asks about *the* gun. Police officers sometimes know what they're asking about. There must have been a gun. You answer truthfully, "Yes, officer, I saw the gun."

Another issue that arises in survey research is *response bias*. Some people will always answer "True" or "Yes" no matter what the question. Other people will always answer "False" or "No." Those of you with small children know some kids answer "No" to every question. There are people who always rate themselves with high scores—plenty of "6's" and "7's." And there are people, modest, self-effacing types, who always rate themselves with low scores—plenty of "2's" and "1's." Well-constructed surveys take response bias into consideration by reversing the wording of questions and by a careful array of questions. So there may be a question, "I find myself getting nervous on a daily basis," coupled with a differently worded question elsewhere in the survey, "I am usually calm, cool, and collected." We would find response bias if the person answered "true" to both questions or gives similar self-ratings.

We've considered issues that complicate the interpretation of surveys—biased samples, the sensitivity of the topic in question, the wording of the questions, and response bias. There is a last issue to consider. It is not an unimportant issue. We need to consider the accuracy or validity of the responses. John says he drinks three beers a day. Does he? Doris says she votes Republican and curls her hair. Does she? Philip says he's chronically anxious. Is he? Betty says she's rarely anxious. Is she?

These are difficult things to find out. Do people do the things they say they do? Or do people tell us what puts them in favorable lights? And do people tell us what they think we want to hear?

A Midwestern university conducted a survey a few years ago about seat belt use. This was a school where everyone drove to and from class. You can imagine the traffic jams. The sociology department asked students in the cafeteria a simple question. "Do you regularly wear your seat belt when you drive?" Almost everyone said they did. The sociology department then stationed observers at the gates to the campus. The observers counted the number of people who wore seat belts. The percentage was less than 60%. Sometimes people do not do the things they say they do. When it comes to the use of seat belts, this discrepancy can have serious consequences.

Incidentally, the routine use of seat belts is a social-cultural phenomenon dating from the mid-1980s. We have to wear seat belts today. I don't know about your country, but in New Jersey it's the law. The police can ticket us if we don't wear seat belts. They have check points on roads in New Jersey where the police look inside cars and see who's belted in and who's not. In the 1980s the use of seat belts was not mandated by law. It's estimated that only 20% of drivers regularly wore seat belts in the 1980s. The other 80% exercised their constitutional right to go head first through the windshield.

The next method I'll like to discuss is called *correlation*. Correlation is more of a statistical technique than a method, but it is so widely used in psychology that we need to treat it as a formal topic. *Correlation is a statistical technique that allows us to examine the relationship among sets of scores.* Correlation does not deal with individual scores but with sets of scores. The sets are called "variables."

The usual procedure is for a group of people—a sample—to fill out two or more surveys. For example, a group of students might fill out a survey about their attitudes towards tests and test taking and a second survey assessing how introverted they are. Every person in the sample fills out both surveys. We then correlate how the two variables are related.

In the old days small samples of participants were studied on a few surveys. Thirty people. Fifty people. One hundred people. Today, the samples are huge and the number of variables large. Computers make that possible. In medical research it's not uncommon to have thousands of participants and twenty or more variables. Computers do the work. Our goof-off time increases. You can do correlations and many other statistics on Excel on your home computer. If you don't have a home computer, you can use the computer at school or on the job.

There are many kinds of correlations depending on the requirements of the sample and the nature of the variables, but all formulas are constructed to produce a score that ranges from -1.00—through zero—to +1.00. There can never be a correlation lower than -1.00 or greater than +1.00. If there is, we can be sure a mistake has been made. There can be a correlation of .00. Usually, we don't say "positive one" and we don't use the plus sign. We usually say "negative one" and we do use the minus sign. And note that we do not use the zero digit to the left of the decimal. It's never "zero point something." It's always "point something."

The range of correlations reflects what you might remember from high school as the number line. You might recollect that you can fold the positive numbers over the negative numbers, using zero as the peg, and come up with exactly the same values. So .73 is the same value as -.73 and -.44 is the same value as .44.

Each correlation coefficient, as the number is technically called, provides two pieces of information. It tells us the *magnitude* or *predictability* of the relationship and it tells us the *nature* or *direction* of the relationship.

Correlation allows an insight into the magnitude or predictability of the relationship among variables. If I know a person's score on survey X, can I predict that person's score on survey Y? If I know your attitude towards tests, can I predict how introverted you are? And if I know how introverted you are, can I predict your attitude towards tests? The answer to these questions depends on the magnitude of the correlation. The closer the correlation is to 1.00 or to -1.00, the greater the predictability. A correlation of 1.00 or -1.00 provides perfect predictability. A correlation of .00 has no predictability. A correlation of .00 indicates that the nature of the relationship among variables is random.

In psychology we rarely get correlations greater than .60. This is not perfect and it leaves a lot of room for uncertainty. But the relationship is not random. A correlation of .60 is better than nothing. I suppose it's at the level of a trend.

The correlation coefficient also provides information about the nature or direction of the relationship. We call any correlation above zero a "positive correlation." We call any correlation below zero a "negative correlation." We call a zero correlation a "zero correlation." It doesn't mind.

In a positive correlation the variables have a *direct relationship*. High scores on one survey are associated with high scores on the other survey. Low scores on one are associated with low scores on the other. If you scored high on the introversion survey, you'll score high on the attitudes toward tests survey. If you scored low on the introversion survey, you'll score low on the attitudes toward tests survey. The variables are like two trains pulling out of a station and going in the same direction. I'm sure this has happened to you. The local you're on pulls aside the express and for a while you see the same faces in the other train. Maybe the faces are laughing at you. Maybe they're blowing you kisses. Eventually, the express pulls ahead and you're left to wonder what that was all about.

In a negative correlation the variables have an *inverse relationship*. High scores on one survey are associated with low scores on the other survey. Low scores on one are associated with high scores on the other.

If you scored high on the introversion survey, you'll score low on the attitudes toward tests survey. If you scored low on the introversion survey, you'll score high on the attitudes toward tests survey. It's like two trains pulling out of a station in different directions. The express is headed uptown. The local is headed downtown. You don't see anyone's face but your own reflection. That's a chance to comb your hair and fix your makeup.

Let me give a few examples of correlations. There's a positive correlation between the amount of time students spend studying and the grades they get on quizzes. The more time students spend studying, the higher they score on a quiz. Conversely, the less time students spend studying, the lower they score on a quiz. Of course, students would like the correlation between study and grades to be a negative correlation. Alas, it isn't.

There's a positive correlation between education and income. The more years of school a person has, the higher the income. This is true in every case but mine.

There's a negative correlation between time spent partying and grades. The more time students spend partying, the lower their grades. Conversely, the less time students spend partying, the higher their grades.

There's a negative correlation between income and playing the state lotteries. The lower a person's income, the more likely he or she is to buy lottery tickets. The higher a person's income, the less likely he or she is to buy lottery tickets. People at the poorest socioeconomic levels play up to fifteen times the number of lotteries as people in the highest socioeconomic levels. Playing so many games of chance may be a reason poor people stay poor. We see them at the bodega counters. I saw one recently. An elderly lady four feet tall. She put her smokes on the left side of the counter. She put her bag of meds on the right side of the counter. She spent the next fifteen minutes ordering lottery tickets and wheeling her lucky numbers. When she was done, she turned and faced me. "Sonny," she said, waving the wad of lotteries, "this is my ticket out of here." I thought, "Fat chance," but I didn't say anything. I didn't want to disillusion her with the odds. Instead of wasting her money playing lotteries she won't win, she should be buying liquor so she can forget she's poor.

Let's look at correlation in the context of television viewing. Grade school and high school students spend an average of six hours a day in front of screens. This includes television screens, computer screens, and whatever other kinds of screens there are. This adds up to forty three days a year—I suppose all this screen viewing prepares children for what they will do in the adult world. The numbers add up rapidly. If we live to seventy five, we will have spent nine years of our lives watching television. That's nine full years. I don't know what else we could be doing with nine full years of our lives.

Television viewing is negatively correlated with lower reading and math scores in grammar school. The more television children watch, the lower their scores on state tests. The less television children watch, the higher their scores. A reason for this may lie in the passive and non-interactive nature of television. Children just lie there and look. What they look at is pretty dumb. If children look at a lot of dumb programs, well, you know what happens.

Television viewing is positively correlated with obesity. One in three American children is overweight. Thirty percent of American adults are obese. Certainly, lying on a couch looking at dumb programs contributes to gaining weight. We don't just lie there. We lie there and munch on snacks. We lie there and sip soft drinks. When it comes to children a key element in obesity may be the advertisements they see. A vast number of commercials in children's programming feature snacks and soft drinks. This advertising is incredibly effective. Children see something in the store and they remember they saw it on television. They see it on television and they search for it in the store.

Television viewing is positively correlated with a tendency toward aggression and with a view of the world that is unrealistic and terrifying. Television portrays a vast amount of aggression and violence. By the time children graduate from high school they will have seen more than eight thousand simulated murders and more than one hundred thousand acts of aggression. Donnerstein and his group watched more than three thousand programs in 1996-97. They found that 60% of programs had violent acts in them and that only 25% of these acts portrayed any sort of moral, legal, or personal consequence. The situation has worsened since Donnerstein's study was published in 1998. The portrayal of violence and of risky behaviors such as smoking, drinking, and promiscuity is nearly as common in PG-13 movies today as it was in R-rated movies in the late 1990s.

Television violence is often pointless. It goes mostly unpunished. It's frequently portrayed as fun and as something cool people engage in. Often, the violence is perpetrated by the hero of the program. We rarely see the perpetrators get caught. We rarely see the implications for the victim or for the victim's family.

There are two concepts that emerge from the study of learning that may help us understand the relationship between television and a tendency toward aggressiveness. These principles are *habituation* and *desensitization*. Habituation involves reduced responding to repeating stimuli. Karl Popper (1902-1994), the eminent philosopher of science, observed that the first time children see violence they are terrified. They run away and hide. But with repeated viewing of violence they are no longer terrified. They stay and turn up the volume. They become desensitized. In desensitization emotions diminish. The fear goes away. Children become acclimatized to violence. Violence becomes the norm. They're no longer upset by images of violence. In fact, it takes increased portrayals of violence to affect viewers. If a character's head doesn't get blown off three minutes into the program, the channel gets changed.

Television portrays a riskier and more violent world than exists. It shows people engaged in destructive behaviors, such as drinking, smoking, dope peddling, promiscuous sex, abusive relationships, and motor vehicle recklessness. It portrays strangers as malevolent, authorities as repressive figures, and serial killers as geniuses who outwit the law between station breaks. I don't know where you want to live, but I don't want to live in the world television offers.

Television viewing at a young age is positively correlated with a later diagnosis of attention deficit disorder. A large study of more than two thousand children correlated the amount of time parents reported their children watched television at ages one to three and a diagnosis of attention deficit disorder at age seven. The more television watched at those ages, the greater the incidence of attention deficit diagnosis. The American Academy of Pediatrics recommends that children under the age of two should watch no television whatsoever. This advice flies in the face of what happens in many homes where the television is on all the time and is used as a baby sitter.

The relationship between television viewing in infancy and a later diagnosis of attention deficit disorder may lie in the timing of brain growth and the nature of television. Infants' brains are growing by leaps and spurts in the first years of life. When they watch television they are exposed to a medium that is rapidly edited. The cameras rarely stay in one position for more than a few seconds. The real world doesn't move the way television cameras move. The real world isn't edited. The real world is ponderously slow and stable. The constant movement found on television may interfere with the ability to concentrate on slower moving events, which is most everything in the real world. Exposed to a rapidly edited medium, children may not tolerate a slower paced version of events.

As you can tell, I'm quite down on television. If we want our children to be ignorant, overweight, and aggressive, let them watch television. If we want our children to be intelligent, buff, and law-abiding, shut the television off and talk to your children. Read to them. Ask them questions. Pay attention to their answers. Challenge them intellectually in ways they can handle. As we will see in the chapter on the brain, this is going to make all the difference in the cognitive development of children. We often look to biology to explain intellectual differences in social class and in ethnic groups. The higher socioeconomic classes are brilliant, the lower socioeconomic classes aren't. These differences may reflect something as simple as shutting off the televisions and talking with children. Hart and Risley (1995) studied forty two families for two years. They sampled the number of words spoken in the homes of professional parents and in the homes of parents on welfare. Children in the homes of professional parents heard an average of more than fifteen hundred words per hour than children heard in the homes of welfare parents.

We don't need electronic gadgets to make our children brilliant. All we need is talk. And talk is cheap.

Correlation is a useful technique in organizing data. A two digit number describes the relationship between scores on surveys. But there is a limitation to correlation that we should always keep in mind. Correlations *describe* relationships. They do not *explain* relationships. Correlations tell us what goes with what. They don't tell us *why* what goes with what.

Consider the positive correlation between obesity and television viewing. It's true that the more hours of television children view, the more likely they are to be overweight. But we cannot conclude that watching television makes children overweight. Nor can we conclude that being overweight makes children watch television. Both are possibilities, but we don't have sufficient information to decide which is the case. A third factor may be causing both television viewing and obesity. This factor may be genetic. Or it may be temperamental, such as activity level. Some children are inherently more active than others. These children like to be up and about rather than glued to cushions in front of television screens.

Consider the negative correlation between television viewing and low grades on state tests in math and English. It's true that the more hours of television children view, the lower they score on state tests. But we cannot conclude that watching television makes children score low on tests. Nor can we conclude that scoring low on state tests makes children watch a lot of television. As with obesity, a third factor may be causing both television viewing and low scores. This factor may be genetic. Or it may be motivational. Some children don't have the skills to master math and English—maybe they had bad teachers.

Correlation is not the same as causation. This is a slogan in psychology. It is a slogan that is often forgotten. You should remember it as you read the text and as you go through your careers. To state cause-and-effect relationships involves acquiring a lot more information than what we usually have available in correlational research.

Consider the following—there is a positive correlation between positive thoughts and the remission of symptoms in diseases. We cannot say that positive thoughts cause the remission of symptoms. It's more likely that the remission of symptoms causes positive thoughts, but we can't say that either. To prove that positive thoughts cause the remission of symptoms involves gathering additional pieces of information. We need to know the incidence of positive thoughts and the worsening of symptoms. We need to know the incidence of negative thoughts and the remission of symptoms. And we need to know the incidence of negative thoughts and the worsening of symptoms.

Consider a related example. Let's say I claim that a particular psychotherapy cures major depression. Before I can claim that with certainty I need to identify the incidence of three other conditions. I need to know how many people got worse taking my therapy. I need to know how many people got better without taking my therapy (or got better by taking a different therapy). And I need to know how many people got worse without taking my therapy (or got worse by taking a different therapy).

In psychology we show a cause-and-effect relationship by conducting an *experiment*. In an experiment *we manipulate one variable to see how this manipulation affects or changes a second variable.*

In life we conduct small experiments all the time. We try a new toothpaste and observe our teeth whiten. We try a new shampoo and observe our hair get fluffier. We try a new skin cream and observe the wrinkles disappear. These substances seem to work. We've proven their effects. But we haven't. Not yet, anyway. Remember what I just pointed out. Before we can claim that we proved a substance works we also need to experience a different substance and no substance. Will our teeth get whiter with a different toothpaste or with no toothpaste? Will our hair get fluffier with a different shampoo or with no shampoo? Will our wrinkles disappear with a different skin cream or with no skin cream?

There are two ways to proceed in experiments. We can use the *pre-and-post test* method or the method of *comparison of groups*.

In the pre-and-post test method I obtain a baseline in some variable in a sample of individuals. How white are their teeth? How fluffy is their hair? How smooth is their skin? I then introduce the new toothpaste or the new shampoo or the new skin cream and observe whether the baseline changes. If these substances have an effect, the baseline should change. If these substances have no effect, the baseline will not change.

To confirm that it is the new substance we introduced and not a different factor that caused the change, I can remove the substance and see what happens to the baseline. If the substance we introduced was the cause of the change in the baseline, the baseline should change again. It should revert back to how it was before the substance was introduced. If the substance we introduced was not the cause of the change in the baseline, the baseline should stay the same.

The pre-and-post test method is a refinement of the *before-and-after* method we frequently observe in weight loss advertisements in the back pages of magazines.

In the comparison of groups method one group of individuals receives the substance under study and a second and comparable group does not. We give one group the new toothpaste, for example. We do not give the toothpaste to the second group. Maybe we give a third group a different toothpaste. We let all the groups brush for a few weeks and then we compare the whiteness of their teeth. If our toothpaste works, the group that used it should have sparkling smiles. The other groups will keep their lips closed and speak with their hands in front of their mouths in order not to be ashamed of their teeth.

An experiment starts with a *hypothesis*. As you recall, a hypothesis is a statement that can be tested. In correlational research a hypothesis involves stating which variables are associated with one another. In an experiment a hypothesis is stated as an "If, then" statement. "If people do X, then Y will happen." "If people do such-and-such, then such-and-such will happen." "If people use this toothpaste, then their teeth will whiten." "If people use this shampoo, then their hair will become fluffy." "If people use this skin cream, then their wrinkles will disappear."

The "if" part of the hypothesis is the "cause." The "then" part is the "effect." In an experiment we are dealing with two broad categories of variables. *Independent variables* correspond to the "if" clause. They are presumed to be the causes in changing behavior. *Dependent variables* correspond to the "then" clause. They are the changes that occur after the independent variable has been administered.

Independent variables correspond to the procedure of the experiment. They are everything the experimenter controls and manipulates. In an experiment the experimenter controls everything—certainly everything he or she thinks may get in the way of the relationship between the independent variables and dependent variables. *Dependent variables are the outcome or result of the experiment.* They are called "dependent" because, ideally, changes in them are exclusively dependent on the independent variables.

The logic of experimentation is quite straightforward. It's so straightforward even the people who live in Astoria can understand it. Experimenters define a class of variables that they can control. They give those variables to one group of people or animals. The group that receives the independent variables, including the key variable that is stated in the "if clause" of the hypothesis, is called the *experimental group*. A second group, called the *control group*, undergoes the same procedures and experiences the same events as the experimental group with one important difference. The control group does not experience the crucial variable stated in the "if clause" of the hypothesis.

Experimenters then define a class of variables that serve as the outcome or result of the experiment. After the groups receive or do not receive the independent variable their performance is compared on the dependent variable. Is the performance of the groups different? If it is, we can conclude that the independent variable changed the dependent variable. That is, the independent variable caused the dependent variable to change. The independent variable had an effect on the dependent variable. If the performance of the groups is not different—if both groups score about the same on the dependent variable—then we can conclude that the independent variable did not cause the dependent variable to change. The independent variable had no effect in changing the dependent variable.

Let's move beyond the level of toiletries and develop an example of experimentation from the realm of memory. I have the hypothesis that *reciting text improves memory for the text*. I almost said recite "out loud," but that would be redundant and repetitive. If people recite text, then their memories for the text improve. I truly believe that recitation improves memory, but just because I believe it doesn't mean it's true. I believe a lot of things that aren't true. The relationship between recitation and retrieval is for research to decide. This is what the empirical method is all about. So I conduct an experiment.

Half the people in this room will recite the first ten pages of our textbook. The other half will read the pages silently. After an hour of reading everyone is given the same multiple-choice quiz covering the first ten pages. If my hypothesis is correct, the group that recited the ten pages will score higher on the quiz than the group that read silently. Maybe my hypothesis is incorrect. Maybe the group that read silently will score higher on the quiz. Or maybe both groups will score about the same.

In this example the independent variable is reciting the text. The dependent variable is the multiple-choice quiz. The experimental group consists of the students who recite the text. The control group consists of the students who read silently.

You're probably thinking that if half the students recite the text, this is going to be a noisy room. The noise level will interfere with studying.

The noise level will confuse the relationship between recitation and retrieval. You are right to think this. But remember the experimenter sets up the procedure. To control for noise level we can separate the members of the experimental group. We can send everyone to different rooms. Or we can conduct the experiment one student at a time.

The bright students are thinking—how does a person get into the experimental or control groups? That's an important consideration and one that brings us to the concept of *randomization*. We want to be sure that every person in the experiment—they are called *participants*; the older term was *subjects*—has an equal chance of getting into the experimental group. We want to pick participants blindly. So the name of every student goes onto a card and each card goes into a hat. We shake the hat thoroughly and pick a card without looking. The first name chosen goes into the experimental group. We shake the hat again and pick another card without looking. This person goes into the control group. We shake the hat again and pick another card—experimental group. We shake the hat again and pick another card—control group. We keep shaking the hat until every person in the class has been assigned to a group. We shake the hat to guarantee that the names don't form a particular order.

Randomization of participants is vitally important in experiments. Many statistical procedures require the assumption of randomization and randomization is a way to prevent bias. We want experimenters to be honest and not to stack the cards in their favor. What if I was an unscrupulous experimenter and I found out that one person in the class was a memory whiz? I might accidentally on purpose put this person in the experimental group. The retrieval of the first ten pages of the book will reflect the whiz's skills and not the overall performance of the experimental group. And what if I was unscrupulous and found out that one person in the class was a clod when it came to memory? I might accidentally on purpose put this person in the control group. The low retention of the first ten pages of the book will reflect the clod's lack of skills and not the overall performance of the control group.

Psychological research employs large numbers of participants because extreme scores obtained by whizzes and by clods have less input in large groups than they do in small groups. I can demonstrate this by income. Most of us probably make around the same income. Let's face it—if one of us was wealthy, he or she wouldn't be here. I know

I wouldn't be here. So everyone in the experimental group is making approximately the same amount of money. Thirty people are in the group. The thirty-first person, chosen randomly, of course, happens to be wealthy. The average income rises substantially and does not accurately reflect the overall composition of the group. Let's change the scenario. We now have three hundred people in the experimental group. All of them make roughly the same salary. The next person selected to be in the group is wealthy. Yes, the average goes up, but not as much as when there were thirty people. The same idea holds if the person was poor. The effect of low income is less significant in a group of three hundred than in a group of thirty.

Let's conclude the experimental method with a second example. I have a new hypothesis—vitamin B12 improves memory. This may or may not be the case. Because I have the hypothesis doesn't make it true. I have to get data, which is what empiricism is all about. I randomly divide half the members of the class to be in the experimental group and half to be in the control group. Members of the experimental group get the independent variable. In this case, they get a thimble filled with a little blue vitamin called B12. The control group gets nothing. Every member of the class silently studies the first ten pages of the textbook. After an hour of study I give out a multiple-choice quiz on the first ten pages. The quiz is the dependent variable. If my hypothesis is correct, the group that received vitamin B12 should retrieve more information and answer more questions correctly. Maybe my hypothesis is incorrect. Maybe vitamin B12 has no effect on memory. Maybe vitamin B12 interferes with memory. In those cases the control group should get more answers correct. Or maybe both groups score about the same on the quiz.

The bright ones in class are thinking, "Wait a moment. This is a bad experiment." The bright ones are right to think that and they're very kind not to express their thoughts for the less bright ones to hear. Just getting a pill—vitamin B12 in this case—may affect behavior and cause a change in the dependent variable. Participants in the experimental group get a pill in a thimble and are asked to read ten pages of a textbook. They are then tested on the pages. Even the people who live in Bushwick will figure out that the pill is supposed to affect memory.

What I need in this case is a second pill and a second control group. The second pill is a *placebo*, which is a substance that has no physiological effect. It's a fake pill. A placebo is needed to control for the possibility that merely getting a pill—any pill—may affect the dependent variable.

I need to start over in a different classroom and randomly select people to be in one of three groups. The experimental group gets vitamin B12 in a thimble. They go off and study the first ten pages of the textbook. Then they come back and take a quiz. The first control group gets a pill that looks like vitamin B12, tastes like vitamin B12, smells like vitamin B12, but is a fake. They go off and study and come back and take the quiz. The second control group gets nothing—we may hand them an empty thimble for a souvenir. Like the other two groups, they go off and study and then come back and take a quiz.

Consider the possibilities. If the experimental group scores higher on the quiz than both control groups, we can conclude that vitamin B12 has a positive effect on memory. If the first control group—the one that took the placebo—scores about the same as the experimental group, we can conclude that vitamin B12 does not affect memory. Rather, it is the act of getting a pill—any pill—that boosts memory. The placebo worked as well as the real vitamin. If all three groups score about the same, we can conclude that vitamin B12 does not affect memory. And we can conclude that in this instance getting a pill—any pill—does not boost memory.

There is another factor we need to take into consideration in experiments. We want the experimenter to be *blind*. This is the idea that experimenters should not know which group they are interacting with. If I know a person is in the experimental group, I may inadvertently look and act differently than if I know a person is in the control group. Maybe I hand the participants the thimble with more authority. Maybe I'm more lively. Maybe I'm more alert. My appearance shouts, "Take your vitamin B12 and see how it improves memory." When I hand the thimble with the placebo to the participants in the control group maybe I do so in a lackadaisical manner. Maybe I'm less lively. Maybe I look bored. My appearance whispers, "Here, take your lousy placebo. It's not going to do anything."

The idea that the verbal and nonverbal behavior of the experimenter may influence the outcome of the experiment sounds farfetched, but we want to consider every possibility. Experimenters may try to control themselves, but we wouldn't want their behavior to affect the participants. Ideally, the people who think up the hypotheses and design the experiment should not be the same people who conduct the experiment. The people who conduct the experiment should not know whether they're interacting with a participant in the experimental or control group.

A word about placebos. They cannot cure disease, certainly not serious diseases, but they have a use in medicine. If the doctor believes a pill is effective, the patient picks up on that belief and rallies. My father was in the hospital some years ago with stomach problems. He asked the morning nurse for a painkiller. The nurse said she'd have to consult with God—she called the doctor. A short time later she came back with a pill in a thimble. My father took the pill and the pain went away. That evening, the pain returned. Pain often comes back in the evening. We don't know where pain goes in the daytime. Maybe it goes shopping. Maybe it takes in a movie. Maybe pain has a part-time job. My father asked the night nurse for his painkiller. The nurse told him he wasn't on a painkiller. My father said he got a painkiller in the morning. "Mr. Ford," the evening nurse said, "that was Tylenol." The pain hurt really bad when my father heard that.

Experiments are the way we show, or strive to show, cause and effect relationships, so they are very valuable in science. It is not always possible to conduct experiments, however. There may be too many variables in a situation and there may be ethical constraints.

Experiments work by controlling as many extraneous variables as possible. They are highly controlled and artificial situations. This is their strength and their weakness. Control and artificiality allow for an arrangement where relationships among causes and effects can be observed in their simplest and clearest condition. I want to find out how recitation affects memory and nothing else. I want to find out how vitamin B12 affects memory and nothing else. To do this, I have to control through my design of the experimental procedure and manipulations everything that may confuse or obscure the relationship between the independent and dependent variables.

Control and artificiality are also weaknesses in experimental research. Real life is cluttered and confused and loaded with God knows how many variables. Think about how you study. Probably, there are a lot of things going on that can affect how you score on the quiz. And think about all the foods you consume while you study. Probably, there are a lot of vitamins churning in your system while you read the text. Probably, there are a lot of other chemicals churning besides vitamins, but we don't want to know about those.

In experiments the relationship among variables is very much a signal-and-noise relationship. The relationship between the independent and dependent variables, if it exists, is the signal. Everything else is noise. We want to create a situation in which the signal can be observed in its purest form. We want to squelch all the noise that obscures the signal. We can't do this in the real world, but we can do it in the laboratory. In the real world signals are hard to observe. But in the artificial arrangement of an experiment the signal may stand out clearly. Or it may blink faintly and for that glint we should thank our lucky stars.

I want to point out that psychologists conduct research—whether case study, survey, correlation, or experiment—under a strict code of ethics. All research is, or should be, peer-reviewed. I could not conduct research secretly and without getting the approval of the social science department and of the school administration.

The code of ethics insists that I do no harm to any participant. I need to obtain what is called "informed consent" before I start. I need to tell the participants everything that is going to happen in the course of the research and why I am conducting the research. The issue of informed consent—in this case the lack of informed consent—has played a controversial role in famous experiments, notably in Stanley Milgram's experiment on obedience, which we cover in the social psychology lecture. In his experiment Milgram misled the participants about the true purpose of the research.

Participants are free to leave the experiment at any time and not complete the procedure. The names of the participants are to be held in strict confidentiality. Participants are to be debriefed at the end of the research and they are to share in any benefits gained from the research, other than in whatever money I earn winning the Nobel Prize.

Thank you.

Tips to Students ~
Tardiness

I'd like to pay homage to Mel Brooks's timeless piece of advice in his comedy classic *The Producers* and alter the line from "Be a smarty and join the Nazi Party" to "Be a smarty and don't be tardy."

It's important that students come to class and that they come on time. Tardiness can be costly. It can result in lower grades. When students are tardy, what do they have to do? They have to ask someone for the notes they missed. How do they know the notes they copy are any good? Maybe the person loaning the notes wrote down the wrong information. Maybe the person started to daydream and missed notes. Maybe the person wasn't on time and was himself or herself tardy. When you copy someone else's notes, you may be copying someone else's mistakes. I don't know about you, but I like to make my own mistakes.

The usual culprit in explaining tardiness is the Metropolitan Transit System. Everybody knows the trains run badly. Miss one and we can file our nails to the cuticles before the next train arrives. The point here is to save your fingernails and your grades. Students signed up for the class knowing what time it started. Presumably, students knew they could make it to class on time.

I once came upon another culprit for tardiness. This was narcissism. A few semesters ago I had a student who was fifteen minutes late to every class. Her name was Candy—that was probably her stage name. She was an exotic dancer. She certainly looked and dressed the part. After the ninth class I worked up the courage to ask why she was chronically tardy. She answered without a trace of shame and pointed to her classmates, "So they can see me."

I couldn't argue with that. I watched her strut to her seat on three-inch heels nine times. Of course, the seat was in the last row on the far side of the room.

I wish I could say Candy got an A in the course, but I can't. Fifteen minutes late for fourteen class periods adds up to a lot of lost notes. I can add that Candy had no trouble getting notes when she asked the men in class—they must not have been good notes.

A last word about tardiness. Tardiness may bring out the entrepreneurial spirit and be a way to earn a few bucks. If a fellow student asks to copy your notes, you should be paid for providing them. It is a loan, after all. I don't know what the rate for copying notes is, but a dollar or two a page sounds reasonable.

LECTURE THREE ~
Memory

I selected memory as the first substantive topic for two reasons. The understanding of memory can assist us in becoming better students. And I think memory is one of the most interesting and important topics.

Our memories may not be the same as our identities, but our memories form the core of our identities. Memory provides the continuity of our existence. I knew who I was when I woke up this morning. I knew what I had to do and where I had to go. Imagine if I had to relearn who I was every morning. Imagine if I didn't know what I had to do or where I had to go. That may sound like a loafer's dream, but it would be quite disconcerting after a while and it would be quite the chore to have to become myself all over again.

It's not only the events of this day. My memories extend backward in time quite a way. They didn't use to, but, alas, they do. And my memories extend forward in time, too. I have memories of the things I need to do tomorrow and the day after that and forward into the faraway future, or so I like to think.

There are many ways to consider memory. We can consider memory *neurologically*, as when the brain ages and when the brain is affected by alcohol and by drugs. We can consider memory *legally*, as in the importance of eyewitness testimony and in jury trials. Often, testimony has to be read back in court because jurors forgot what was said. We can consider memory *scholastically*, as in its importance in the education system. We can consider memory *psychotherapeutically*. It's a central theme of many therapies that people become psychologically disordered when they forget experiences or motivations. And it's another central theme that people regain their psychological health when they recover the memories of these experiences or motivations. We can consider memory *interpersonally*, as when one spouse remembers instructing the other spouse to bring home rye bread and gets pumpernickel instead. I'm sure many family spats involve memory.

We can consider memory in a *social-cultural* context. Many memories are shared among groups. Consider what happens when retired jocks get together and reminisce about their high school football team. Mention the game with Alfred Smith High and everyone remembers with glee the details of that crushing victory. Mention the game with Michael Bloomberg High and everyone remembers with regret the details of that crushing defeat.

Consider the events of September 11, 2001. People remember shared experiences of that terrible day. I once heard a radio discussion whether the events of September 11, 2001, would be remembered on September 11, 2101. The consensus among the guests was—that depends on what happens in the intervening century. I'm not sure that answer is correct. Terrible events that affect an entire nation can be forgotten. The greatest catastrophe ever to befall America was pretty much forgotten until the recent fear of bird flu restored it to our collective consciousness. I refer to the flu pandemic that occurred in 1918 and killed in one year as many Americans as died in the four-year-long Civil War. I suppose I can understand why *The Spanish Lady*, as the flu was called, was forgotten. We may not consider dying on a battlefield as particularly glamorous, but it's more glamorous than dying of influenza.

In this lecture we consider memory *psychologically*, perhaps with a dash of the scholastic sense sprinkled in for flavor. In the psychological sense memory is defined as *the persistence of learning and of experience over time*.

In psychology memory has been studied in the subfield of experimental psychology. The study goes back to the founding of psychology. *Herman Ebbinghaus* (1850–1909) was a German who studied memory in the 1880s and whose book *Memory: A Contribution to Experimental Psychology* has stood up well across more than a century. Many of Ebbinghaus's conclusions are still in the textbooks and are considered fundamental phenomena of memory.

Ebbinghaus used himself as a subject. He created lists of *nonsense syllables* that he memorized under controlled conditions. He also tested himself on the recall of these syllables to examine forgetting. A nonsense syllable is a three letter, consonant-vowel-consonant, combination, such as TOX, DEL, BIJ. Ebbinghaus created nonsense syllables because he believed that memorizing lists of words would be too easy.

Memory is enormously persistent and comprehensive. Think of all you know and for how long you know it. If we took all my memories, put them in boxes, and trucked the boxes across the Verrazano Bridge, all the people living in Staten Island would have to move to accommodate the space required to store the boxes. And if you boxed up all the memories I forgot and trucked those to Bayonne, all the people living there would have to move to make space.

With respect to capacity, has anyone ever reached the limit of memory? Well, there was that guy who frequented the bowling alley, but it's not proper to talk about him. And with respect to the temporal persistence of memory, consider elderly people who recollect events that occurred decades previously. My grandfather told me a memory of an event that occurred in Ireland eighty years previously. It seems a cow stood on the foot of a peasant and refused to budge. Cows weren't bright in the Ould Country in that time period. Neither were the peasants.

Memory is certainly impressive. So is forgetting. One of my themes in this lecture is that *memory is fragile*. We forget all the time. We misremember all the time—I remembered pumpernickel and she was sure she said rye. We forget important events in our lives. We forget entire chunks of our lives. Try to remember events from grammar school. We were alive then and full of memories on a daily basis, yet we can retrieve only a few scattered events. The vast number of daily memories has taken up residence in that overpopulated land of oblivion.

We forget important events and we remember things that never happened. In her autobiography *Shelley Two* the actress Shelley Winters writes of being home on November 22, 1963. She writes that she was watching television and saw President Kennedy get assassinated. Unless Shelley was part of the conspiracy, that never happened. Shelley refers to the Zapruder film, the horrible movie that shows the assassination. The Zapruder film was not shown on television until 1971, eight years after the assassination. What Shelley did is common. She misremembered events and combined two memories into a coherent recollection. One recollection was of watching television in 1963. The other recollection was of watching television in 1971. The two memories fit together snugly and the combination was plausible. But events did not happen the way Shelley recollected that they did.

Memories are fragile, even memories hoary with age. Our memories are not copies of events, they are *constructions* or *reconstructions* of events that have happened or, as when we remember the future, of events that have not yet happened.

I very much want to disabuse students of the notion that human memory works like a camcorder or like a computer disk. Far from it. Human memory does not resemble camcorders or computer disks. Human memory is *limited, selective, emotional*, and *changeable*.

Camcorders and computer disks provide us with *verbatim memories*. They capture a full recording of whatever is put on them. And they do not contain emotions. I walked from the train station to this classroom. I'm sure I passed people. I have no recollection of any of the people I passed. Maybe I would have some recollection if they had been especially attractive or especially appearance challenged. If I wore a camcorder around my neck I would have a complete record of everyone I passed. The images would not change over time—maybe the colors would fade, but nothing else would change. I can put the camcorder in a closet and take it out after ten years and play it. Nothing would have been added. Nothing would have been erased. That's not how human memory works. After ten years memories would have changed. After ten years most faces would have entered oblivion. And if the memories were important perhaps a face or two would have been added that were not part of the original memory.

Similarly with a computer disk. I'm typing a term paper and accidentally type two periods after a sentence. I put the disk in the same closet as the camcorder and let ten years pass. Nothing on the disk is going to change. The second period is going to be there. That's not how human memory works. After ten years the second period may have disappeared. Or maybe a third period is added or one of the periods changes into a comma. Our memories are changeable.

We might expect small and unimportant memories to change. Large and important memories change, too. There's a category of memory called *flashbulb memories*. Flashbulb memories are formed when we encounter unanticipated and emotionally-wrenching experiences. An example is remembering where we were when we heard about the attack on the World Trade Center. For students who are old enough, another example is remembering where they were when they heard that the *Challenger* space shuttle exploded on lift off. For students who are still older, another example is remembering where they were when they heard President Kennedy was assassinated. We might expect these searing memories to be fixed in neuronal concrete, but they are not.

Ulric Neisser, an important memory researcher, had his general psychology students write down their memories learning of the *Challenger* explosion the day after it happened. Two years later he located forty four students of the original class. He asked the students to recall their memories learning of the *Challenger* disaster. Eleven students gave completely inaccurate accounts. Their second recollections did not match the original recollections written the day after the event. Only three students provided recollections that matched the original memories. The majority of students recalled a mixture of accurate and inaccurate details.

Before we move onto the memory model I'll like to touch on the *accuracy of memory*. This is an important topic and one that is difficult to ascertain given that memories are selective and changeable. Accuracy plays an important role in the legal justice system. There are people on death row solely on the basis of eyewitness testimony. We hope that eyewitnesses are certain of what they saw, but confidence in one's memory is no guarantee that eyewitnesses truly saw what they remembered seeing.

Similarly, accuracy of memories became an important issue in the 1980s and 1990s as psychotherapists conjectured, falsely as it turned out, that mental disorders were based on forgotten (repressed) memories of traumatic abuse in childhood. This conjecture led to the "memory wars" between psychotherapists, who based treatment on the recollection of trauma, and experimental psychologists, who suggested that recovered memories were false memories created in the process of psychotherapy.

Accuracy is of fundamental concern, but it is extraordinarily difficult to ascertain. Consider witnesses who, without any corroborating evidence, say they saw such-and-such happen. Consider troubled people who, without corroborating evidence, claim they were abused by relatives in childhood. The past is gone and leaves few traces. Most of the time there is no objective evidence beyond fragile memory to identify the truth of events.

The rare occasions when corroborating evidence exists hardly support the notion that memories correspond with events. Shelly Winters wasn't accurate. Nor was John Dean. Dean was President Nixon's lawyer back in the time of the Watergate scandal in the early 1970s. Dean became convinced that Nixon was setting him up as the fall guy in the scandal. Dean wasn't going to fall for that and jumped ship. He testified before Senator Sam Erwin's committee and was soon entitled the "human tape recorder." I suppose if he testified today we'd call him the "human voice-activated recorder." Dean seemed to possess a verbatim memory of events in the Oval Office. He seemed to recall everything that was said, literally word-for-word.

A little later another employee named Alexander Butterfield jumped ship. Everyone was jumping ship by this time. They figured the Nixon administration was going to join *Titanic* on the North Atlantic seafloor. Butterfield testified to the Erwin committee that Nixon bugged the Oval Office and was recording what was said. Once the Supreme Court ruled that Nixon had to surrender the audiotapes of the bugging it became possible to compare what Dean said was said in the Oval Office with what was actually said. Dean was not the "human tape recorder." He was the "human mis-tape recorder." He got the *gist* of what was said, but hardly word-for-word. Contrary to the impression he made, he was wrong about many of the details.

With respect to the accuracy of memories, it is important to distinguish between the *personal truths* of memory we carry around in our heads and the *historical truths* of events as they actually occurred. Memories are not copies—I remember saying this previously. Memories are the narratives or stories we tell ourselves about events. They are not the events themselves. If we're fortunate, personal truths correspond with historical truths. Often, we're not so fortunate and the two do not correspond. The personal truths we possess may be self-satisfying. They may be self-glorifying. They may be self-deluding. We have to be careful that personal truths do not replace or distort historical truths. The disconnection between personal truths and historical truths can have grave consequences, as in the legal justice system and in psychotherapy.

I'll like to outline the *memory model* introduced by Richard Atkinson and Richard Shiffrin in 1968. Research has moved beyond the memory model and has seriously complicated it, but the model remains a useful way to organize our thinking about memory.

The memory model consists of three processes. These processes are encoding memories, storing memories, and retrieving memories.

In the process of encoding information gets into memory. For example, encoding the information for a quiz or encoding the names and buying habits of customers. For another example, encoding what we did during summer vacation.

In the process of storing information stays in memory. The notes students studied have to stay in memory long enough for them to take the quiz. The names and habits of customers have to stay in memory long enough to make the sale. And the events that occurred during the summer vacation have to stay in memory long enough to prevent the lawsuit.

In the process of retrieving memories get out of memory when they are needed. The notes have to come out of memory and be available when students take the quiz. The customer's name and preferences have to come out of memory and be available when she walks in the store. And the events that occurred in summer have to come out of memory and be available when the police knock on the door.

I'll like to take a stroll through the garden of the memory model and review a few phenomena associated with each process. We can start with encoding.

Most information gets into memory through *effortful encoding* or *elaborative rehearsal.* Certainly, most of what goes on in the education system involves effortful encoding. We think about what we have to memorize. We study the information and ruminate over it. We ponder the information and contemplate it. We don't simply repeat the information in a rote manner, we elaborate on the information. Sometimes we lovingly dote on the memories and sometimes we hate to review them. Repetition may be the mother of memory, but it is always more than simple repetition that goes on cognitively.

Ebbinghaus discovered what is bad news for students—the news hasn't improved since the 1880s. *There is a positive correlation between encoding and retrieving.* The more effort we put into encoding, the more likely we are to retrieve the information when we need it, such as when we take a quiz. Studying takes time. Studying takes effort. We can't place the books on our foreheads and expect intellectual osmosis to occur. To the contrary, study is work. Sometimes it's hard work. Make sure when you study that you place pillows on the floor. In the event you pass out from all the hard work studying, you won't hurt yourself.

A few weeks ago I stopped in the library. The librarian was in a panic. A student was bent over a textbook and smoke was coming out of her ears. The librarian wanted to sound the alarm and summon the fire department, but I saw what was occurring before a false alarm was sounded. The student was making such an effort studying, her brain had caught on fire. The smoke was venting through her ears.

Ebbinghaus discovered what can be good news for students—the news hasn't dimmed since the 1880s. *The more we know about a topic, the easier it is to learn something new.* Conversely, the less we know about a topic, the more difficult it is to learn something new. The study tip is obvious. It's important that students apply themselves at the start of the semester. The first few chapters may be difficult, but it gets easier as the semester progresses. Some students—badly misguided students—coast for the first few weeks and do not apply themselves. They realize in the middle of the semester that they're in danger of failing. They hit the books. The books hit back. These students have no background in the material. They start reading the middle of the book. They've missed a lot of information in the first half of the book. They have to start cold. That is not an easy thing to accomplish.

Ebbinghaus discovered that people encode information more effectively if they study in short segments and repeat the information frequently. This is entitled the *spacing effect* or *distributed practice* and it compares favorably with *massed practice*, which is also known as *cramming*. Many students study in one long session the night before a quiz. They burn the midnight Con Edison in the attempt to make up for lost study time. Cramming is an inefficient and self-defeating way to study. Cramming leads to poor long-term retention of the information and it places a lot of stress on the student in the study session. It's one thing to study for an hour. It's another and stressful thing to study for four hours. As we shall see in the lecture on sleep, the loss of sleep may reduce memory for the same information that kept us up. Sleep plays an important role in consolidating and preserving memories.

A better way is to study in short intervals. I can't recommend an exact period of time, but half an hour or forty five minutes sounds reasonable.

Study for this amount of time and then do something else, preferably not something intellectual. As we shall discover in the section of this lecture on forgetting, an intellectual task may retroactively interfere with the information studied. Do something non-intellectual. Jog. Shoot hoops. Talk on the phone. Listen to music. After a while, return to the study—but be sure to review the notes made before you took the break. Distributed practice is effective because it reduces stress and it increases repetition of information.

Ebbinghaus discovered the *serial position effect*. He discovered that he remembered the *beginnings and ends of lists* of nonsense syllables better than he remembered the nonsense syllables in the middles of the lists. The serial position effect is a common phenomenon. Consider this example. It's the first day on the job and the boss introduces our co-workers. There are twelve people standing in a semi-circle. He starts, "Meet Mike, Jack, Betty ..." and he concludes with "...Rudy, Tim, and Tom." If we're like Ebbinghaus, we remember the first few names and the last few names. The names of the co-workers introduced in the middle of the list—persons four through nine—are a babble and a blur.

Consider this example. Our significant other calls and lists a number of grocery items we should buy on the way home. The list starts with apples and ends with zucchini. The items in the middle of the list? They're a babble and a blur. We stop at the local supermarket. We're okay with apples and zucchini, but not with anything else. We buy the wrong items. We miss items. I think our significant other should have done the shopping. And I think there's going to be an argument when we arrive home.

There's a study tip involving the serial position effect. Put the most important items at the beginning or end of the study session. Don't bury the important material in the middle. To do so is to maximize interference from other memories. And if we have a quiz, we should study for the quiz last and then go to bed.

There's another kind of encoding or processing. This is *automatic encoding*. It's precisely what it says—information gets into memory automatically and without rehearsal. I don't doubt that important information slips into memory automatically, but many automatic memories involve the incidentals of our experiences. For example, remembering the picture that was on page three hundred of the textbook. When students read and think about page three hundred, the picture should be last thing on their minds. But inexplicably the picture gets into memory, quite as if it was as important as the text.

Perhaps I shouldn't downplay automatic encoding. We rely on it when we try to find lost objects. "Where are my car keys?" we ask excitedly. "Where's my cell phone?" "Where's my wallet?" To answer these questions we revisit our behaviors and mentally trace where we were. We didn't pay attention to the detail of placing our car keys somewhere. We didn't memorize where we last made a call. We didn't rehearse laying our wallet down. We hope, desperately, that the information slipped in automatically. If it didn't, we're rather in trouble.

The question now is—what do we encode? What do we store?

We don't encode a verbatim rendition of events. Memory is limited and selective—I'm sure I said that. *We encode what we think about.* Encoding involves elaborative rehearsal. It's not enough to repeat information in rote fashion. That may or may not work, but it's a dull way to do business. A better way to encode is to take what we need to know and hook it up with what we already know.

Encoding involves elaborately rehearsing the *meaning of events or of information.* There's an important study tip here. We'll encode information and successfully retrieve it if we find a meaning for it in our lives. Students should try to personalize the topics in a course. "What can I use here?" "How can this help in my life?" I tell the kids, yes, geometry is a boring subject, but you have to get a passing grade in the course. Yes, geometry is dull, but it can come alive if you derive a meaning for it. If a kid was artistic I stressed the usefulness of geometry in art—the table in Da Vinci's *Last Supper* is a straight line. If a kid liked baseball, I stressed how he could learn geometry in terms of baseball. A shot down the right field line is one kind of angle. A shot up the middle is another kind of angle. A shot down the left field line is a third kind of angle. A shot that goes backward over the head of the umpire is a foul tip.

Memory is not verbatim. We encode the *gist* of things. Recall John Dean of Watergate fame. He got the gist right. He got the particulars wrong. When we go to church, we don't recall the homily verbatim, not unless the minister said something clever or cracked a joke from the pulpit. Instead, we recall the gist of the sermon—he preached about eternal damnation.

We encode *images* or mental pictures. Generally, memory for pictures, such as for faces, is superior to memory for verbal information. Years ago, Allan Paivio, a Canadian psychologist, found that people tended to remember concrete nouns better than they remembered abstract nouns. Paivio used a procedure in verbal learning called *paired associates* to demonstrate this effect. A paired associate is a stimulus-response combination, such that when the stimulus word appears we're supposed to say the response word. For example, when we hear "orange," we're supposed to say "sand." When we hear "justice," we're supposed to say "hope." Paivio found that concrete stimulus-response paired associates such as "orange-sand" were recalled more reliably than abstract stimulus-response paired associates such as "justice-hope." He conjectured this occurred because it was easier to form a mental image of a concrete paired associate than it was to form a mental image of an abstract paired associate. It's easier to form an image of an orange lying in sand than it is to form a mental picture combining justice and hope.

There's a study tip here. To maximize storage and retrieval we should strive to make what we have to memorize as vivid as possible. We should strive to use as many senses as possible. "John Watson was a tall man." "His hair was white." "He spoke with a gruff Southern accent." "He walked heavily." "He smelled of cheap cigars."

Paivio suggested there were two encoding systems. One is *visual*, as when we form images. The other is *verbal*, as when we memorize the abstract words that reference numbers and facts and theories.

We also encode on the basis of *sound*. Everyone on Jerome Avenue in the Bronx has experienced the *tip-of-the-tongue phenomenon*. People who don't live in the Bronx have experienced it as well. We know that we know something, we even know that it starts with a particular letter, let's say with "D," but we can't recall the specific item. Maybe we retrieve it at a later time—"Dion DiMucci"—but the memory gave us the slip when we needed it. Probably, we retrieve it on the drive home and hours later.

We can combine meaning, imagery, and sound into the idea of story telling as a memory aide. If we want to remember something, we can make it into a story. We can create characters to carry the concepts we're trying to memorize. We can add conflict and controversy to the story. We can spice it up with color and with vivid images. And we can shape it so it has a beginning, middle, and end. Story telling is a venerable way to memorize things. It does not guarantee high grades, but it's a fun way to study.

In the early 1970s Fergus Craik and Robert Lockart introduced the concept of *levels of processing*. This concept has somewhat faded from the books, but the idea is relevant to what I've been trying to get across. The deeper and more thoroughly we process information, the more likely we are to store and retrieve it. In their research Craik and Lockart flashed words on a screen for one second. Participants in group one were asked to pay attention to whether the words were in capital letters. Participants in group two were asked to note if the words rhymed with a test word. Participants in group three were asked to identify if the word fit in a test sentence. After the list of words was presented, all participants were asked to recall as many words as possible. This request came as a surprise, since they were not asked to do this at the start of the experiment. The dependent variable was the number of words recalled. Participants in group three recalled the most words. Participants in group one recalled the least. Craik and Lockart suggested this occurred because participants in group three had a more complex task that involved processing or analyzing the words in greater detail than the participants in groups one and two. Their conclusion restates the concept of elaborative rehearsal. The more we mentally elaborate on a task, the more likely we are to retrieve it. The more superficial the elaboration, the less likely we are to retrieve it.

Let's move onto the second step in the memory model—*storing*.

There is a transitory and complete storage at the level of the senses. Perhaps this occurs as sensation transforms into nervous transmission. The original discovery was made with vision and is called *iconic memory*. A researcher named George Sperling flashed a stimulus array of letters to participants for a fraction of a second. The array consisted of three rows of three letters. Think of seeing the eye chart in an optometrist's office. When asked, participants could remember the items in the top row—this is the serial position effect at the level of the senses. When Sperling unpredictably cued the second or third row by placing an arrow next to it, participants could retrieve the items on that line successfully. Sperling reasoned that there was the briefest verbatim image of the array, otherwise the participants would not retrieve items from the second or third rows. Remember that the array flashed for less than a second. And Sperling reasoned that the participants were not reading the array. They didn't have sufficient time. They must have been getting a complete image.

Sensory storage is fascinating, but it is not what most people think of as memory and it is observed only with the use of specialized equipment. When most people think of memory, they think of the widely known terms short-term memory (or short-term storage) and long-term memory (or long-term storage).

Short-term memory is a brief, limited, and easily disrupted memory system.

"How brief?" you ask. Unless rehearsed, information deletes from short-term memory within one – twelve seconds. I say "one second" because we've all had the annoying experience of forgetting a thought instantaneously. I say "twelve seconds" because of an important experiment by Margaret Peterson and Lloyd Peterson in 1959. They gave participants nonsense syllables to keep in memory and then asked the participants to count backward by three from a number for a particular period of time. After the period of time elapsed, participants were asked to state the nonsense syllables. Retrieval of the nonsense syllables served as the dependent variable. For example, a participant was given the nonsense syllable SUL and asked to count backward from six hundred eighty seven for nine seconds. The logic was that counting backward would prevent rehearsal of the nonsense syllable and interfere with retrieval. The logic was right. After only three seconds counting backward, retrieval of the nonsense syllables was on average 80%. Counting backward for nine seconds resulted in an average retrieval of 40%. Counting backward for twelve seconds resulted in an average retrieval of 20%. Note the difference between 40% retrieved and 20% retrieved is a paltry three seconds. What can a fellow do in three seconds? Not retain nonsense syllables, apparently.

Over the years there have been a lot of variations on the Peterson and Peterson study. The conclusion is that loss of information from short-term storage depends on the number of items held in storage and on the number of disruptive items more than it depends on the mere passage of time.

Short-term memory lasts for a brief amount of time. Short-term memory is also limited in capacity. "How limited?" you ask. Short-term memory is limited to *five-to-nine pieces of information.* In the old days the term was five-to-nine *"chunks"* and a grand term it was. We like to think we have unlimited cognitive capacity. Alas, we don't. I understand the current emphasis is on multi-tasking. This is something we're not very good at, despite what we tell ourselves. Five-to-nine chunks—the average is George Miller's famous "magical number seven plus or minus two"—doesn't offer a lot of cognitive room to multi-task in.

I suppose there are countless examples of short-term memory and of its duration and capacity. We've all had the experience of thinking about one thing and having a new thought pop the first thought into the side pocket of oblivion. The classic example is what use to happen in phone booths. Today, if I want to make a phone call I reach in my pocket, take out a gadget, and start talking. In the old days I had to go to a place called a "phone booth." Young people may not know what a phone booth is. There aren't a lot of them left, not in the sense of having glass doors that closed and offered privacy. There are, of course, public phones, but they're not enclosed and they don't offer privacy.

Let's say that back in the day I want to order pizza on my way home. I find an uninhabited phone booth, get my quarter out, and deposit it in the slot. I dial the operator for information. "Hello, can I have the number of Vinnie's Pizzeria on Kennedy Blvd.?" "Sir," the operator replies, "that number is 420-0418." At this instant I have a memory problem. I have to keep repeating (rehearsing) "420-0418" while I retrieve my quarter and dial Vinnie's for a pie topped with sweaty pepperoni.

Consider this possibility. The quarter doesn't return and I have to fiddle through my pockets for another coin—I really want pizza. Five seconds pass. Ten seconds pass. Twenty seconds pass. All the while I have to keep repeating "420-0418." Maybe I ask myself where the quarter is. If I do that, I just put myself in trouble. The question is like the three digit number in Peterson and Peterson's experiment. "42—oh, what's Vinnie's number?"

Consider this possibility. The operator answers my question and gives me Vinnie's phone number. But it's not "420-0418." "It's 420-041873220167892." This number exceeds the five-to-nine item limitation of short-term memory. Looks like I'm not having pizza tonight.

I mentioned that short-term memory is easily disrupted—is "disruptable" a word? Peterson and Peterson's experiment demonstrated that. And my phone booth example can demonstrate that. I get my quarter back, place it in the slot, and start to redial. At this moment a man excitedly knocks on the door of the booth. "Hurry up!" he yells. "I need to use the phone. My wife is having a baby." "One moment, please," I reply, "I'm ordering pizza. The number is 42—oops." The man distracted me and the number bounced into the side pocket.

Before I leave this example let me advise how we can avoid the limitations of short-term memory. Rather than repeat "420-0418," I can *write the number down*. Writing it down makes the number permanent and frees up memory. I can rehearse the items on the next quiz rather than Vinnie's phone number. Writing our thoughts keeps us from forgetting them. I can refer to the written record whenever I want to order pizza.

I knew a psychologist who believed creativity was precisely this process of making short-term memory permanent. He believed that everyone—maybe we should qualify this and say most everyone—thinks creative thoughts—puns, wordplay, insightful observations, and the like. We no sooner think something creative than something else—a non-creative thought, shall we say?—pours into our minds and distracts us. After the distraction we want to reclaim the creative thought, but it's been oblivionated. As the song goes, the creative thought is "lost and gone forever." If we write the thought down, we don't lose it. We capture impermanence on scratch paper.

Short-term memory and long-term memory are separate memory systems. Short-term memory can with some leeway be conceptualized as the doorway to long-term memory. We rehearse chunks, we elaborate on them, and they become more permanent. *Long-term memory is a more permanent memory system.* It is immense in scope, it lasts indefinitely, and it is not so easily disrupted. Note, however, that long-term memories can and do change. And they fade over time.

Sometimes a distinction is made in long-term memory between *recent memories*, such as for the events that occurred last week, and *remote memories*, such as for the events that occurred in childhood.

Long-term memories are categorized in different buckets or boxes. Every sense involves memory—as we shall learn in the lecture on the brain, this involves association neurons. I haven't smelled a particular odor for years, but I smell it now and I instantly know what it is. I haven't heard a particular lyric for years, but I hear it now and I instantly know the name of the song. I haven't seen a particular place in years, but I see it now and I instantly know the name of the street.

Semantic long-term memories involve memories for facts and for information. Semantic long-term memory involves memories for verbal information—for anything we can put into words. "Albany is the capital of New York." "George Washington was the first president." "Seven times seven equals forty nine." "The Bronx is up and Staten Island is down."

We carry in our minds a vast array of reference materials—we're walking, talking, and breathing reference libraries. Word books, dictionaries, thesauruses, atlases, encyclopedias—they're inside us. We're a Google and a Wikipedia unto ourselves. The education system can be conceptualized as a gigantic project in which students acquire semantic long-term memories. This project starts in kindergarten and it ends— we like to think it never ends.

Information in semantic memory is impersonal—knowing Albany is the capital of New York floats in the neuronal ether outside the particulars of my life—and it rarely has a connection to time or to a personal narrative. Most semantic memories exhibit what's called *source amnesia*. We rarely remember when we acquired particular semantic memories or who taught them to us. Pertinent to my example, I invite students to try to remember when and where they learned that Albany is the capital of New York.

Autobiographical or *episodic long-term memories* involve memory for the experiences of our lives. Autobiographical memory is the story of my life. It is, as it says it is, my autobiography or personal narrative. I know what Coney Island is and where it is—these are semantic memories. I remember going to Coney Island last August and riding the Cyclone and eating a knish at Nathan's on the Boardwalk—these are autobiographical memories. I know that George Washington was the first president—this is a semantic memory. I remember visiting his mansion at Mount Vernon, Virginia, and pocketing some of the silverware—these are autobiographical memories.

Autobiographical memories are, obviously, personal. They involve things we do. They involve things that happened to us. They are connected to particular people and places. They are connected to specific sources. And they are related to time in a direct way. I arrange the events of my life in chronological order. Grammar school came before high school. High school came before college. College came before unemployment.

Autobiographical memories are called *episodic* because we don't remember every detail of our lives. We remember a few episodes or incidents that are arranged in chronological order. We don't remember every event in grammar school or high school or college. We remember a few events that stand out for whatever reason.

Few people remember events that happened before the age of three. When they occur, such memories are like snapshots rather than coherent episodes. They might be considered the trailers rather than the movies of our lives. This failure to remember events so early in life is referred to as *infantile amnesia*. There are a number of reasons for this. The brain may not be sufficiently mature. Children of these years are learning to process and utilize language—so much of our memory involves words. Finally, children may not know how to properly encode and store memories—these are tasks some college students haven't mastered.

This is not to say that children under the age of three lack memories. They remember Mom. They remember Dad. They remember Uncle Dennis. They remember games. They remember the last time they played a game with Uncle Dennis. But such memories do not survive. They are rarely recalled when the children grow up.

There's a third category of long-term memory. This is *procedural long-term memory*, which is memory for nonverbal bodily and muscular processes, such as skating and skateboarding and surfing and driving and keyboarding. Such processes depend on muscular movements. None of them depend on words. In fact, adding words to procedural memories can cause mishaps.

Consider the last two. We can't tell ourselves in words how to drive. We can only get behind the wheel of a car and drive. If we go into a skid, we can't remind ourselves to "Take my foot off the gas pedal and drive into the skid." If we tell ourselves that, we'd crash before reaching the end of the sentence. We can't tell ourselves in words how to keyboard. We can only keyboard. If we're typing an essay, we wouldn't get far if we had to hunt and peck for letters. "Now, where is that 'G' key?" "Where is that 'Y' key?" "Where is that dern 'B' key?" Experienced keyboarders type without looking at the letters. Experienced keyboarders know they made a mistake merely by the motion of their fingers.

Let's move onto *retrieving*, which is the process of getting information out of memory when we need it. Retrieval is the dependent variable in the memory model. It is the test of memory.

There are three ways retrieval is assessed. These ways are the recognition test, the recall test, and the relearning test.

In the *recognition test* of retrieval people have to indicate whether they have seen a particular item before. That is, they have to indicate whether they recognize an item. The item is present. It is in front of them. They have to indicate if they recognize it. They have to pick the item out.

Police lineups and photo arrays involve recognition. The suspect is standing in a group or his mug shot is included in a collection of photographs. Witnesses don't need to send a bathysphere into the hadal depths of memory. The suspect is standing in front of them. They simply need to pick him out.

Multiple-choice quizzes are tests of recognition retrieval. The question on the quiz is:

Wilhelm Wundt believed psychology was the study of:

    a)   the conscious minds of normal people
    b)   the unconscious minds of abnormal people
    c)   observable behavior
    d)   none of the above

To answer this question we don't need to rent a submersible and descend into the deep-sea trenches. The answer is staring us in the face. "Pick me, pick me!" choice a) is crying. All students have to do is recognize the choice. The answer is not in the students' minds. It is on the paper squirming in frustration that it's not recognized.

In the *recall test* of retrieval we need to load up on canisters of oxygen and rent submersibles. In the recall test we are given no information. We must retrieve all elements of the memory. From scratch, so to say, and on our own.

Describing a perp—a perp is, but you already know what a perp is—to a police sketch artist involves the test of recall retrieval. We have to supply all the details. The perp is not physically present. "He had a brown suit on," we tell the officer. "He was tall. He had red hair and freckles and a third eye in the middle of his forehead." I tend to think this perp won't be hard to catch.

Essay quizzes involve tests of recall. In an essay quiz students are handed a paper with this question, "What did Wilhelm Wundt believe psychology should study?" Under the question is a blank piece of paper. The answer is in our minds. We better set sail and find it or our grade is going to sink.

Students often believe that essay quizzes are easier than multiple-choice quizzes, but that's not so. Probably, what is easier is the grading of the types of quizzes. Answers are black and white on multiple-choice quizzes. There are shades of gray in answering essays. Professors sometimes pass shoddy work on essays with the attitude that students knew what Wilhelm Wundt believed psychology should study, but just can't express themselves. Multiple-choice quizzes are easier because half the students' work is done. The answers are provided for them. Students simply need to recognize the answer.

Relearning is the third test of retrieval. In relearning students are asked to learn the same material a second time. Maybe they've forgotten the material. Maybe a period of time has passed, such as the time between the fall semester when a person failed a course and the spring semester in which he or she repeats the course. The finding with relearning is that the material is more quickly learned and subsequently retrieved the second time compared to the first time.

If I may be permitted to self disclose, something I do only about topics to my credit, I took four years of Spanish when I was in high school and college. I could read Spanish fluently. I read *El Diaro*, the Spanish daily. I read Cervantes. I read Borges. I never needed a dictionary. I never needed to look a word up. I could read Spanish fluently, but I couldn't speak or understand a word. Conversation skills were not taught in those days.

Life has moved on and those literary bilingual days are long past. I know so little Spanish today, *ay Dios mio*, I can't read the advertisements on the subway. Here's the point with relearning. If I were to go back to school and take Spanish up again, I would learn it—relearn it—rapidly. Perhaps more rapidly than I learned it the first time.

We might conclude that the second course refreshed long dormant vocabulary words. Maybe the words were reposing in the brain's sub-basement. Maybe they were in a hemispheric bunker in the Thunder

Mountain of my mind. This conjecture sounds plausible, but it is difficult to test. We would have to control for the possibility that I'm a better student today than I was back in the day. Maybe I pick Spanish up more rapidly the second time not because the neuronal cobwebs are dispersing, but because I'm a better student. And we would have to control for motivation. Maybe I pick Spanish up more rapidly the second time because I'm more motivated than I was the first time.

I'll like to cover two important processes involving retrieval. Before I do, I'll like to insist that the likelihood of retrieval depends directly on the extent of encoding. If I encode something thoroughly and deeply, there's a good chance I'll retrieve it when the time comes. If I do a poor job encoding something, there's an equally good chance that I won't retrieve it when the time comes. This is true of the names of co-workers. This is true dealing with customers. And this is true taking quizzes.

The first important retrieval process I'll like to describe is *mood-congruent retrieval*. Information and events encoded in a particular mood are more easily retrieved when in that mood. So information encoded when we are sad will more easily be retrieved when we are sad. Events encoded when we are angry will more easily be retrieved when we are angry.

Mood-congruent retrieval plays a crucial role in anger and in interpersonal conflict. This is a point I'll explain in the lecture on emotion. To anticipate—we get in arguments with our significant others. When we get angry we remember all the other times he or she made us angry. We start arguing over the milk I failed to bring home. (Milk was buried in the middle of the list rather than at the beginning or end.) Before we know what happened, we're arguing about something that happened in the past. She remembers all the other groceries I failed to bring home. I remember another topic that made me angry—not the milk, but the milkman.

When we slip into particular moods the events encoded in those moods return into awareness. We remember events experienced while in a particular mood. Our significant other makes us angry—we retrieve memories of all the other occasions he or she made us angry. Our significant other makes us sad—we retrieve memories of all the other occasions he or she made us sad.

New York people are a particularly dour group. If I ask one to tell me a joke, I get swearwords instead. So I'll tell a joke to New Yorkers. It's a Benny Hill original, so don't blame me if you don't laugh. "A ship carrying red paint crashed into a ship carrying blue paint and the survivors were marooned." The joke makes you laugh. It fills you with happiness. And it restores memories of jokes that made you happy in the past. It puts you in the mood to tell me a joke in return.

Mood-congruent retrieval demonstrates an important memory principle—*what we retrieve depends on our current emotional state.* We're angry—we remember angry events. We're sad—we remember sad events. We're in love and we're filled with the rosy glow of happy memories about our dear beloved. We fall out of love and we're filled with a different set of memories. The memories aren't so rosy now. They're a morose shade. What do we now remember about the other person? What do we say about the other person when we fall out of love? "I didn't think she was that kind of person." "I didn't think he was that kind of person."

The second important retrieval process is *context-dependent retrieval.* This is the situation in which encoding and retrieving get commingled, such that it is possible to retrieve memories only when we are in the same situation in which we originally encoded them.

Context-dependent retrieval sounds exotic, but it is a common occurrence. And it is a phenomenon that bears directly on studying. Let me give three examples.

Let's say we return to the town where we grew up. We haven't been there in years. We hardly remember the place. But when we return and walk around the old neighborhood we are flooded with memories. "There's the candy store Charlie use to run." "There's the house where George and Robbie lived." "There's the building where Kay and Jerry lived." We are overwhelmed with memories. We retrieve the memories in the places where they were encoded. We would never retrieve them if we didn't return home.

A person witnesses a crime. But he can't remember a single detail. So the police return him to the scene of the crime. He walks around and the details of the crime come back into memory. "Now I remember. The perp ran out of Hamburger Haven and crossed the street in the direction of Manhattan Books." We're confident that New York's Finest will soon collar the perp. The city can stand down.

I don't know how often police return witnesses to crime scenes, but if I were a judge I wouldn't allow that procedure in my courtroom. It's too easy for the police to manipulate recollections as the witness walks around the crime scene. "The perp ran out of Hamburger Haven and went in the opposite direction from Manhattan Books." The detective frowns and shows disapproval. The witness notes this and changes the story. "Wait a moment, officer, the perp ran out of Hamburger Haven and crossed the street in the direction of Manhattan Books." The detective smiles and expresses approval.

The third example of content-dependent retrieval concerns studying. It never fails that after a quiz a student will say she studied a lot but bombed on the quiz. "I'm sorry," I say with great sincerity and I ask, "How did you study?" She tells me. "I study by lying in bed in my pajamas, smoking, snacking, and listening to Barry Manilow love songs." Well, that explains it. The information in the textbook got linked to the bed, to cigarettes, to snacks, and to Barry Manilow. The student arrives on quiz day wearing clothing. She takes the quiz in an erect seated manner. There are no snacks present and no cigarettes. Barry Manilow is on tour somewhere. The student can't remember anything.

There's an important study tip involving context-dependent retrieval. Students should study in the same way they take the test. Ideally, students should study in the same room and in the same seat. This is not always possible in a crowded college that holds class around the clock. But it is possible to avoid stimuli that might snare the information. Don't study in bed. Don't snack while studying. Don't smoke while studying—it's amazing how many memories get attached to cigarettes. And no music, not even Barry Manilow.

Students can make context-dependent retrieval work for them rather than the other way around. I recommend the following. Suck on a particular mint while studying psychology. Spearmint, how about? Suck on spearmint only when studying psychology and on no other occasion. If you get stuck while taking the quiz on which founder believed psychology should study the conscious minds of normal people, you can't light up a cigarette. You can take out a spearmint and the answer will immediately come to you. "Wilhelm Wundt!" Keep sucking and you'll get an A on the quiz.

Another technique to make context-dependent retrieval work for you is to use a particular cologne or perfume only when you study psychology. Guys can use Aramis. Gals can use Chantilly. If you get stuck while taking the quiz on which founder believed psychology should study the conscious minds of normal people, you can't take out a cigarette. You can raise your soaked sleeves and sniff and the answer will immediately come to you. "Wilhelm Wundt!" Keep sniffing and you'll get an A on the quiz.

This sounds suspicious, but it works. At this point in the lecture I use to take out a travel bottle of cologne and spray my sleeve and pronounce "Wilhelm Wundt!" I no longer do that. It happened one semester that a student had an asthma attack after I sprayed. Maybe I went a little thick with the spray. Maybe I should have bought an on-brand rather than an off-brand.

Smell is intimately related to memory and vice versa. Think how Proust's novel starts—the narrator smells the odor of the Madeleine cookies his mother use to bake. The memory trail ends seven novels later. Maybe you've had the experience of smelling the cologne or perfume your Ex use to wear. A lady smells Aramis and her knees buckle. A man smells Chantilly and his heart races. Raul, a ladies man I knew in college, advised us bush-league Lotharios to wear Old Spice when we went clubbing. Raul claimed the aroma would make women remember their fathers and want to go out with us. I'm not sure of the logic here, but Raul was a successful womanizer. And he must have been a closet Freudian. For most women memories of their fathers are sweet. Perhaps I should say bittersweet. I always worried a woman would smell the Old Spice I splashed on and start shrieking because of her painful memories, "Daddy, please stop! Daddy, stop hitting me!" The possibility of that happening was remote, but that was the kind of luck I had when I went clubbing in college.

Before we move onto forgetting I'll like to cover *mnemonics*, which are *ways to organize encoding in order to make retrieval more likely*. Mnemonics require memorization in their own right. They've got to be created and practiced in order to work.

A commonly used mnemonic is an *acronym*, which is a word or phrase culled from the first letters of other words. There's "Every good boy deserves fruit." The first letter of each word denotes a letter of the music scale. There's "Homes," which is the acronym for the Great Lakes—Huron, Ontario, Michigan, Erie and Superior. "On old Olympus towering top, a French and German brewed some hops." The first letter of each word in this acronym pertains to one of the twelve cranial nerves. And there's "Never eat slimy worms," which stands for the four points of the compass. If people need an acronym to retrieve the four points of the compass, they must be hopelessly lost.

I'll like to describe an interesting mnemonic entitled the *Method of Loci*. The story goes that in the B.C. period a righteous Greek named Simonedes was at a dinner party. The guests were making fun of Zeus. Word went up to Mount Olympus that jocular comments were being made about the god of thunder. This did not go lightly on Mount Olympus. Zeus instructed Simonedes to frequent the outhouse a moment before the roof collapsed, flattening all the guests to protoplasmic anonymity. Fortunately for the mortician Simonedes was a memory expert. He was able to recall the places where each guest sat when the roof fell in. The burials went smoothly.

The Method of Loci requires us to memorize a series of fixed places that we can visit in a sequence. In our imagination we insert the new items we need to memorize at each place in turn. Ideally, we want to make both the places and the items as vivid as possible—you may recollect that concrete items are retrieved more easily than abstract items.

I went to school in the Bronx. I haven't been in the Bronx since 1987. I assume it's still there. If someone stole the Bronx I'm sure I would have heard about it. The mayor would have been on the news asking whoever took the Bronx to please give it back, no questions asked. Anyway, after a few years of hard traveling on the IND line I realized the D train was a mnemonic. It runs the same route on every trip. I can still picture the route after all these years. Fordham Road, for example, was a two-level station with three tracks. The middle track never seemed to be used for anything other than for garbage. I like to think the city has cleaned up the station by now.

Each stop on the D train can serve as a fixed place in the Method of Loci. There's Fordham Road, 183rd St., Tremont Ave., 175th St., 170th

St., 167th, and all the way down to 34th St. where I exited and ran like the dickens to catch the PATH train to escape to the safety of New Jersey. I have no idea where the D train runs north of Fordham Road or south of 34th St. I'm sure there are nice stops along the way, I just never visited them. If I had, my mnemonic would be longer.

Let's say we have to memorize the names of the Roman Caesars. Maybe we're taking a course in Ancient History. Actually, I chose this example because we know how the Caesars looked and acted—most of the time it was not to their credit. We can memorize the list through the bull-headed process of rote memorization, but that wouldn't be any fun. A better way to memorize the list is to utilize the Method of Loci and place a Caesar at each stop on the D train.

The first Caesar was Julius. He was a baldheaded man who was deaf in one ear. In my imagination I can place a baldheaded man with a hand cupped to his ear asking for directions at the Fordham Road station.

Augustus was the second Caesar. He looked like the newsman Ted Koppel or, should I say, Ted Koppel looked like him. In Rome there's a famous statue of Augustus wearing a breastplate and holding a spear. I can ride to the next station and place a Ted Koppel look-alike in a breastplate and holding a spear standing at the 183rd St. platform.

Tiberius was the third Caesar. He was the Caesar when Jesus was on earth. He was the oldest and meanest man in the world. He was left-handed and strong. It was said he could crush an apple in his bare hand. I tried that last night and my hand's been hurting all day long. I can ride to the next station and place an old mean-looking man at the Tremont station. He's standing there and turning an apple into juice. The juice is streaming down his hairy forearm. I can hear the juice drip on the platform. Drip, drip, drip. The juice makes a puddle. I can see the drops bounce upward before they land and stain the pavement. It's like a special effects scene in a horror movie. You may think I'm overdoing this, but the more vivid I make the image, the more likely I am to retrieve it.

I can do this with the rest of the Caesars—I'll run out of stations long before I run out of Caesars. Whenever I need to retrieve the names of the Caesars I can pay my fare and take a ride on the D train.

Let me give another example of the Method of Loci. The great thing is that we can use the same mnemonic over and over. Maybe my memory task isn't as exotic as memorizing the names of long-gone despots. Maybe it's as banal as memorizing the list of groceries my significant other narrated over the cell phone. "Eggs, milk, salami," she starts, concluding eighteen items later with "a six pack of Corona Light." Like she has to remind me about a six pack of Corona Light. The first seventeen items? I could try to memorize them using rote memorization, forcibly rehearsing each item. If I have pen and paper and aren't driving, I can write the list down. Or I can take a ride on the D train. I can place a carton of eggs at the Fordham Road station. To make it vivid, I can crack a few on the pavement. I can place a carton of milk at the 183rd St. station. I can open the carton and spill a little. I can place a package of salami at the Tremont station. I can allow a mouse to open the package and pilfer a slice. And so on down to 34th St., where I can twist open a Corona Light and toast Simonedes for making this possible.

If memory is the persistence of learning and of experience over time, then *forgetting is the loss of learning and experience*. When forgotten, learning and experience go into oblivion, that vast country located to the east of Lithuania.

Forgetting is ubiquitous. It happens all the time and everywhere. It's happening right now in Brooklyn and in the Bronx. New Jersey's not exempt. Neither is Virginia or Utah or Texas. Forgetting isn't limited to the United States. Forgetting is an international phenomenon, just like soccer and professional wrestling.

We forget incidental things. Things like the names of co-workers and of customers. Things like the names of relatives. Things like the names of singers and actors. We forget the lyrics in songs, the names of books, and the characters in books. Professors forget the names of students. Students forget the names of professors—I get called "Mister" on many the occasion. Students forget to do their assignments. Professors forget to grade the assignments. Students forget what they studied last semester. Students forget what they studied last night. We forget to make credit card payments. We forget whether we locked the door to our apartment. We forget whether we shut the coffee pot off. We forget where we put things. We forget why we walked into a room. We forget what we were looking for. We forget whether we performed a particular task. We forget where we put our wallets and cell phones. We forget what we wanted to tell a person. We forget whether we said something. We forget what we were just talking about. We forget where we parked the car and whether we turned the headlights off. We forget whether we left the child in the back seat—we better not forget that.

We not only forget incidentals, we forget entire chunks of our lives. How many memories do we have before we were five years of age? Not many. I was alive when I was nine and there were three hundred sixty five days in that year, but I'm hard pressed to retrieve many memories. It's the same when I was nineteen. It's the same when I was twenty nine. It's the same when I am thirty nine, which is my current age. I suppose I could reconstruct what I was doing in those years, but it would not be the same as specific autobiographical memories.

Forgetting is ubiquitous and instantaneous. Ebbinghaus did carefully controlled experiments involving nonsense syllables. He memorized a list of nonsense syllables to perfection and then tested himself every hour to see how many he recalled. This produced the *forgetting curve*. He found that he forgot most of the nonsense syllables shortly after memorizing them. For example, after nine hours he failed to recall 40% percent of the list.

Some people demonstrate remarkable capacities for semantic memory. Most of us do not. These people seem to recollect a vast number of facts. They are DNA-barcoded encyclopedias. Possibly, they're trying out for quiz bowls or for *Jeopardy*. Perhaps they demonstrate a quirk of brain anatomy. Perhaps they use mnemonics. Perhaps they're highly motivated. They are called "mnemonists" and not infrequently wind up on the stage. Jerry Lucas, a New York *Knicks* forward, was such a person. Maybe the most famous mnemonist known to science was a Russian called Mr. S. His real name was Solomon Veniaminovich Shereshevski, which is why he's called Mr. S.

Other people demonstrate remarkable capacities for autobiographical memories. They seem to recollect everything that ever happened to them. Recently, an American woman named Jill Price published the story of her life. She remembers in detail everything that she ever did or had happen to her since 1980, when she was fourteen. She remembers down to the detail of what she ordered for dinner on a particular day. Remembering every meal we had for decades adds up to a cookbook of autobiographical memories. William James, the influential psychologist and pragmatic philosopher, wrote that if we remembered everything we would be as bad off as if we remembered nothing, but Jill seems not to be bothered by the vast quantity of her memories.

The phenomena of complete semantic and autobiographical memories points in a broad way to why forgetting is ubiquitous and necessary. To function in the here and now, we don't need to retrieve everything. Consider my trek from the train station to the classroom. I passed many people. Some were walking by themselves, as I was. Some were walking dogs. Some were walking babies in strollers—these were usually young fathers. This is a social-cultural phenomenon found in Lower Manhattan. The yuppie fathers appear to baby sit and push the strollers on weekends. I don't know where the yuppie mothers are. Maybe they're at the hairdressers. Maybe they're having their toenails manicured. But back to memory. Unless the people I passed were special in some way, there's no reason to store memories of them. Unless something happened—*memorable*, we say—there's no reason why I need to encode a memory. Encoding everything chokes memory lane with weeds rather than with flowers.

Why would we want to retain all our memories? Sure, we'd like to rehearse all the successes and all the compliments, but there are a lot of experiences that aren't successful and merit accusations. Would we want to remember all the events in which we failed and came up morally short? Would we want to remember all the bad and shameful events? All the events in which we committed sins of commission and omission? All the events in which we were taken to task? I know I wouldn't and I suppose that's why I've forgotten so many things.

We can conceptualize forgetting in terms of the memory model.

We forget information and events because we *failed to encode* them. We did a poor job studying. We didn't pay attention. We were distracted. We didn't engage in effortful processing. We didn't elaborate the material. The information and events never got into memory.

We forget information and events because we *failed to store* them. They got into memory, but didn't stay in. They're unavailable for whatever reason. You might recollect my self disclosure about reading Spanish. I could read Spanish fluently at an earlier point in my life. At this point in my life I can't read headlines. The information was there once of a time. It's no longer there. Where it went to, I can't say. Maybe it's in neuronal bondage somewhere in the brain. Maybe it has joined the ever-lengthening procession into oblivion.

Storage does not directly correspond with the *use / disuse* of particular memories. We've all had experiences in which a memory we frequently access—say a customer's name—is no longer available. It's giving us the slip. And we've all had the opposite experience. Sometimes we recollect a lot of information about a topic we haven't considered in a long time. This happens to me when I notice the obituary of a baseball player. I haven't thought about the player in years—probably, I haven't heard the name in years—but I recollect his team, his statistics, even the number on his jersey. I haven't used the information in a long while, but it comes back quite as if I thought about it on a daily basis.

Finally, we forget because we *failed to retrieve* the information or the experiences. They got in, they stayed in, but they didn't come back when we needed them. This happens to salespeople on a regular basis. They know that they know the customer's name, but they can't think of it at the moment. This happens to students on a regular basis. They know that they know who Wilhelm Wundt was, but they can't remember what he thought psychology should study. This happens to professors on a regular basis. Students say hello and greet them, but for the life of them the professors can't retrieve the names of the students or the semesters they sat in class.

One of my themes in this lecture is to insist that long-term memories can and do change. With respect to the failure of retrieval there is an old theory in psychology called *interference theory*. This is the concept that long-term memories can interfere with one another, thereby complicating retrieval. Similarly, long-term memories can blend with one another, also complicating retrieval. This happened to Shelly Winters when she wrote her autobiography.

There are two types of interference—proactive interference and retroactive interference.

Proactive interference is the phenomenon in which old memories make it difficult to retrieve more recent memories. You might think of the terms "proactive" and "proceed," as in "Let us proceed from the past into the present."

So we know the number of Vinnie's Pizzeria—420-0418. But the number changes. It's now 652-9342. The next time we want to call ahead for a pepperoni pie we can't recollect the new number. We dial the old number. Maybe we dial a blend of numbers—420-9342.

I'm dating myself by the use of phone numbers. Because of cell phones, no one memorizes numbers. We program them into the phones and press a button when we need them. If we need to, we can reprogram the number. Cell phones simplify everything. They also complicate things when they get lost. If that happens, we're not having pepperoni pizza today.

Perhaps a contemporary example of proactive interference involves usernames and passwords. I had a username and a password, but Windows made me change it. Next time I want to go to a particular website, I can't remember the new username or password. I type the old username or password. Maybe I type a blend of usernames and passwords.

Of course, we can write these things down—we better remember where we keep the list.

Here's another example. Last semester I took Spanish 100. This semester I'm taking Italian 100. Every time I try to translate a word into Italian, the Spanish version pops into my head.

The overall logic in proactive interference is: first memorize topic A; then memorize topic B; try to retrieve topic B.

Sometimes this happens. A guy has a former girlfriend. Let's call her "Betty." They break up and Betty assumes the unenviable role of an Ex. The guy has a new girlfriend. Let's call her "Tess." He slips and accidentally calls Tess "Betty." Maybe this happens in a moment of passion. Maybe not. Whenever it happens, Tess is not amused. She's highly insulted. The guy is in danger of assuming the role of an Ex. If this happens to any of the men in class, don't panic. Explain to your girlfriend that the slip up in names is due to proactive interference and is nothing intentional. Of course, she won't believe you, but you have to make the attempt.

Retroactive interference is the phenomenon in which new memories make it difficult to retrieve old memories. You might think of the term "retroactive pay"—pay for past work, which can be quite lucrative. In the case of retroactive interference the present—newer memories—intrudes on the past—older memories—making retrieval more difficult.

We've learned Vinnie's old phone number—420-0418. We've also learned Vinnie's new number—652-9342. For some reason we try to recollect Vinnie's original number. Maybe we see a number and think it's Vinnie's old number. The new number interferes with the retrieval of the old number. Maybe it produces a blend of the two.

We have similar experiences with our usernames and passwords. The new usernames and passwords interfere retroactively with the old usernames and passwords. It's a common occurrence that a username or password doesn't work. We start fishing in memory for an old username or password. Maybe the old ones will work. But we can't recollect the old usernames or passwords because of retroactive interference.

This semester we're taking Italian 100. Last semester we took Spanish 100. Someone asks us to translate a word into Spanish, but we can't recollect the word because of the retroactive interference of Italian.

The overall logic in retroactive interference is: first memorize topic A; then memorize topic B; try to retrieve topic A.

Our guy is with Tess. Maybe it's a moment of passion. Maybe it's not. Whatever the moment, Tess asks if he remembers the name of his previous girlfriend. He doesn't recollect the name because of new learning—Tess has sent Betty into oblivion. I can advise the men in class that if this happens don't tell your girlfriend that you can't retrieve the name of your previous flame because of retroactive interference. Tess thinks it's true love. And that's all she has to know.

There's an obvious study tip involving interference theory. Never study similar topics—psychology / sociology; Italian / Spanish—back to back. Doing so maximizes interference. We always want to separate similar topics. For example, study psychology first, then algebra, and then sociology. And take plenty of breaks in between.

Here's another study tip. Study what you are going to be quizzed on last. Doing so minimizes interference. Study for the quiz and then do nothing intellectual. Watch a movie. Groove to Barry Manilow on the treadmill. Go to bed. If you engage in intellectual work after studying for a quiz, you maximize retroactive interference.

Forgetting happens on a daily basis—no, on an hourly basis, if not on a minutely basis. There is another and more profound form of forgetting. This is called *amnesia*. Unlike ordinary forgetting, amnesia involves the loss of large amounts of memory and cannot be attributed to the memory model. Amnesia results from *trauma* to the brain or to *traumatic events* that affect personality and the mind.

Trauma or traumatic events can result in retrograde amnesia or in anterograde amnesia.

When *retrograde amnesia* occurs the person *cannot recall events that happened before the trauma.* This happens with the proverbial blow to the head that blurs memory for events that happened before the blow. For example, in a car accident the driver cannot recollect where she was driving to after she struck her head against the dashboard. In a football game a player cannot recollect events of the game that occurred before he suffered a concussion.

When *anterograde amnesia* occurs the person *cannot recall events that happen after the trauma.* The person cannot learn anything new.

A famous case study who for decades was known as Mr. H.M. tragically epitomizes anterograde amnesia. Mr. H.M.—his name was Henry Molaison and he died at the age of 82 in 2008. (The names of cases can be revealed after they die.) As a young man Henry suffered from uncontrollable epilepsy. The medications that were available at the time were not successful in reducing the seizures. Based on whatever flimsy evidence was available, the decision was made to operate on Henry's brain. On 25 August 1953 lesions were made on both sides of Henry's brain. The lesions destroyed the right hippocampus and the left hippocampus, as well as adjacent brain sites. The hippocampus is an organ of the brain that, among other functions, converts verbal short-term semantic and autobiographical memories into long-term memories. The surgery reduced the seizures. It also left Henry in a permanent present tense. He could never learn anything new that involved words. He would read the same magazine over and over—each time it was a new experience. He would be introduced to a person. So long as he kept the person in sight, he remembered the person. But if the person walked out of the room and immediately returned Henry would have no recollection of having met him or her. They would have to be reintroduced. This happened if he met the same person day after day.

I'll like to pause for a moment and indicate the tragic and complex nature of this case. The surgery was successful in controlling the epilepsy, but it left Henry in an unenviable state for the rest of his long life. It's difficult to say which problem was worse and which outcome was better. Henry lived without seizures and without the ability to form new memories. His memory stopped the morning of 25 August 1953. It's not very difficult to say that the operation was a case of medical hubris—"experimental surgery" we can call it. The surgeon had no idea whether the outcome would work and he had no idea what he would destroy or what state Henry would be in after the operation. He was operating in the dark and in ignorance. Of course, that didn't stop him.

When amnesia results from brain injury the person loses both autobiographical and semantic memories. The loss of memory is for events that occurred around the time of the trauma—recent memory and not remote memory. Afterward, retrieval for these memories is quite difficult, if not impossible.

Amnesia that does not result from brain injuries is called *psychogenic amnesia*, a condition much popularized in psychodynamic literature and in any number of television movies. You know the plot. A lady is found wandering on a beach. She can't remember who she is or where she's from. Psychogenic amnesia involves autobiographical memories and does not ordinarily involve semantic or procedural memories. And psychogenic amnesia does not usually involve anterograde amnesia. The loss of memory is both for recent and for remote memories. The lady can learn new facts—she's in Keansburg in Monmouth County, New Jersey—and she remembers the English language and how to perform arithmetic. She can ride a bicycle and drive a car. The lady doesn't remember what she did the day before she was found on the beach. Nor does she remember any details of her adolescence and childhood.

Unlike with amnesia that results from brain injuries, autobiographical memories usually return in cases of psychogenic trauma. In this movie the memories return to the disappointment of the lifeguard who fell in love with the lady. She turns out to be Mother Superior of an order of cloistered nuns.

I'll like now to turn to a consideration of *eyewitness testimony*. I do so for two reasons. Eyewitness testimony plays an important role in convicting felons. It also plays an important role in convicting people who are not felons and who are mistakenly identified. And eyewitness testimony demonstrates the fragility of long-term memories. As I've indicated throughout, long-term memories can and do change.

Eyewitness testimony is a powerful and persuasive—a convincing and convicting—type of evidence. We've seen enough episodes of *Law and Order* to know the verdict "Guilty" lights up the jurors' eyes when the eyewitness is asked to point out the perp in open court. Jurors do this because they believe that memory works like a camcorder or computer disk. Jurors fail to appreciate the changeability of memories and the corruption—the corrupt-ability—of memories. Jurors believe memories are complete and verbatim. This belief is false. Jurors believe that memories are accurate and correspond to events. This belief is false. Jurors believe that the expressed confidence of witnesses in the accuracy of their memories is an indication of the accuracy of the memories. This belief is false. Confidence is not an indicator of accuracy.

Jurors are not usually sensitive to police interviewing techniques or to the powerful techniques of coercive persuasion that can distort and even create memories. Detectives and district attorneys are trained interrogators. They are not kindly interviewers. They are not our friends. Their purpose is to close a case and get a conviction. Their purpose is not necessarily to get to absolute truth, a place as distant as absolute zero. They bring powerful interrogation techniques to people who may be vulnerable to manipulation and who may be in dire circumstances.

Contrary to what we see on television, eyewitness testimony is problematical and error prone. People misremember. People remember events that didn't happen. People remember details that are plausible in the context of the crime, but didn't actually occur.

In a review of two hundred twenty four wrongful convictions, one hundred seventy two (77%) were cases of mistaken eyewitness testimony. Mistaken eyewitness identification accounted for more causes of wrongful convictions than all the other categories combined. Wrongful conviction for whatever cause is a serious matter. Innocent people lose chunks of their lives in jail and the real criminal is at large and free to commit other crimes. When it comes to eyewitness testimony, the United States Supreme Court has ruled that a person can be convicted of a major crime (murder, rape, kidnapping) solely on the basis of eyewitness testimony and with no other evidence. Innocent people can spend time—they can spend years—in jail with no other evidence against them than what a witness says.

I defined memory as the persistence of learning over time. Let me give another definition of memory, one that demonstrates the fragility of memory more than its permanence or accuracy.

Memories are the stories we tell ourselves about the things that happened to us.

If we interpret memories as stories and as story-telling, the emphasis on permanence and on accuracy vanishes. We can appreciate that the details of stories can change. Details of stories can be lost—stories are not photographs and do not capture a complete (verbatim) version of events. Details can be added to the stories that were not present in the original telling. The nuances of stories can change depending on the audience. I tell stories differently to my drinking comrades than I do to my parish priest.

An event—a crime—happens one time. Everything after is subject to the principles of memory (and to other factors, as well). I witness a crime. A few minutes later a police office shows up and asks, "What happened?" I retrieve the details of the crime—I tell the officer a story. Retrieving a memory—telling the story—is an act of encoding. The story may change in the telling. A few minutes later a reporter runs up and asks, "What happened?" I retrieve the story and re-encode it. Later, a book publisher calls me. I retrieve the story and re-encode it. Later, I'm in court and the district attorney asks, "What happened?" I retrieve the story and re-encode it. Maybe while I'm waiting in court I hear other witnesses tell their stories of the crime. Maybe I compare my story with theirs. Maybe their stories have details that are lacking in my story. Maybe I add these details to my story, such that when I answer the district attorney I tell a different story than what I started out with. This practice is called *post-event information* and it can have devastating consequences for the legal system. In former days witnesses sat in the same room during trials and were free to talk among themselves. They were free to compare what we might call the "notes of memory." Let's hope this practice isn't allowed in our day. Of course, witnesses were able to talk among themselves before the police and reporters arrived on the scene. And witnesses are free to buy the local newspaper and read about the crime, but only if they hand the sales clerk money.

The underestimation by jurors and police of the factors that can corrupt memory may be changing, at least in the country of New Jersey. In June, 2010, a special master assigned to the New Jersey Supreme Court recommended that eyewitness testimony be treated as *trace evidence* comparable to DNA and to fingerprints and to bullets. Police have to be careful that they do not contaminate eyewitness testimony by violating any of the principles established in more than a century of the experimental study of memory. To avoid contamination of evidence police have to minimize post-event information. They have to take care to prevent witnesses talking among themselves and comparing stories. They have to take care that they limit the information they provide witnesses—it not infrequently happens that police provide details of the crime the witnesses they are interviewing do not know. Police have to take care to prevent witnesses from identifying the same person twice. In this case witnesses may select the suspect the second time out of familiarity rather than from his or her involvement in a crime.

I'll like to review a few factors that make eyewitness testimony unreliable. In the first place eyewitnesses are being asked to do what most people do not do—*pay attention to events*. Eyewitnesses are asked to make judgments about events that may be beyond human capacity to discern. Was the car that struck the pedestrian going forty miles an hour or forty five miles an hour? Was the paper bag Lee Harvey Oswald brought into the Texas School Book Depository the morning of President Kennedy's assassination thirty four inches long or thirty eight inches long? We just don't pay close enough attention to such things and we may not be capable of making such judgments even if we paid attention.

Ordinarily, we go through life in a daze. Mentally, we are someplace else. Crimes like auto accidents and assassinations occur instantaneously. They're over before we know they began. They're over before we know what occurred. We are asked to consider an event that's concluded. We are asked to provide details of an event we paid scant attention to.

When it comes to being in a daze consider the experiment by Daniel Simons and Daniel Levin in 1997. A researcher stops students on a campus and asks directions to a particular building. In the middle of the conversation two men rudely pass between them carrying a door that momentarily blocks the researcher from view. I don't know, maybe the men carrying the door are Laurel and Hardy. As the door passes between them, the researcher steps away and is replaced by a different person. Seven of the fifteen participants in this experiment did not react to the change. Afterward, they admitted to Simons and Levin that they did not notice the replacement. They were surprised to learn the person was different. Strangely, the eight participants who said they noticed the switch continued to give directions, quite as if nothing unusual had happened.

There are *situational factors* involving the crime scene to consider in evaluating eyewitness testimony. Is the lighting sufficient for witnesses to observe events? Are there echo effects? Is a gun present? The presence of a weapon reduces facial recognition—witnesses are looking at the gun rather than at the face of the gunman.

There are *sensory factors* to consider. What are the visual and the auditory capabilities of witnesses? Many people wear eyeglasses that are out of date. This may affect the perception of events at the fringe of vision, say a hundred or a hundred fifty feet away.

There are *personality factors* to consider. Are witnesses motivated to help the police or to feel that they are acting in an important way? There is an extensive literature about people who volunteer in situations— come forward as witnesses—and people who don't volunteer. People who volunteer may tell an interviewer what they think he or she wants to hear. Is the witness prejudiced against a race or a religion? A prejudiced person may see skin color as darker than it is. Generally, people are better at identifying individuals of their own race than of a different race.

There are *cognitive factors* that may affect testimony. If two unrelated events occur close together in time and place, they may be construed as a single event. And they may be construed as related, perhaps as cause and effect.

The *wording of questions* may affect the conclusions witnesses make about events. The wording of questions may affect memories of the events, causing witnesses to insert things that were not present in the original incident. Elizabeth Loftus was a pioneer in the study of eyewitness testimony. In an experiment performed with John Palmer in 1974 she showed students a film of a car accident. The film turned the students into eyewitnesses. Half the students received a survey with a question worded, "How fast were the cars going when they *hit?*" The other half of the students received the survey with the same question worded, "How fast were the cars going when they *smashed?*" Changing "hit" into "smashed" increased the speed of the car. The average estimated speed in the group that read the word "hit" was thirty four miles per hour. The average estimated speed in the group that read the word "smashed" was forty one miles per hour. A week later Loftus and Palmer distributed another survey assessing the students' recollections of the film. This survey included a question asking, "Did you see any broken glass?" Fourteen percent of the group who read "hit" reported seeing broken glass on the pavement. Thirty-two percent of the group who read "smashed" reported seeing broken glass. It's plausible that broken class would be on the pavement after a car accident. There was, in fact, no broken glass.

The procedure in the broken glass experiment demonstrates the pernicious effect of *post-event information* on eyewitness testimony. Post-event information is the situation in which *witnesses retroactively incorporate details in their memories they did not originally experience but found out afterward.* For example, a witness may read a detail in the newspaper or hear it on television. Maybe a witness spoke to another witness or to a police office. Maybe a lawyer mentioned the detail. Whatever the origin, the detail is incorporated into the witness's story quite as if it was always present and experienced at the time of the crime.

Loftus entitles this the *misinformation effect* in her experiments as she adds false details that were not part of the incident (film of the accident). However, witnesses may learn details that were physically present in the incident. Such details are not misinformation but factual post-event information.

The experimental procedure involving misinformation is to present a film of an incident to participants and to ask questions on a survey about the incident. On a follow up survey half the participants are asked about details that were not part of the original incident. Such details are called *intrusions*. The intrusions are quite plausible in the context of the incident—broken glass following a car crash. Half the participants read questions that accurately match the incident and do not include intrusions. Additional surveys can be given out in which both groups are asked about the occurrence of intrusive details. The recollections among participants are compared. Is the group who received misinformation on the second survey more likely to include intrusions in their stories about the incident than the group who did not receive the misinformation? As you might predict, they are more likely to include such intrusions.

The great thing about using students in general psychology classes as participants in research is that the students are trapped. Loftus can administer surveys throughout the semester and see how the misinformation effect plays out. In fact, it becomes stronger as the interval lengthens between the film and the various surveys. Repeated questioning about false details makes such details more likely to be included in the recollections of the incident. If participants are asked once about broken glass they may not be impressed. But if participants are asked multiple times about a detail, they may get the idea that the detail was actually present in the film. After all, the people who made up the survey must know what they're asking about.

The potency of post-event information cannot be overlooked. It is difficult to change the memory of an event that was successfully encoded. It is not so difficult to change the memory of an event that was poorly encoded.

If I saw the suspect wearing a blue jacket, it is difficult to convince me that he wore a red jacket. If I did not notice the color of his jacket, it may not be difficult for me to add the color red into my story when I find it out later. This detail adds color to the story, but it can be bad news for the suspect if a red-colored jacket was erroneous at the outset. I may say the jacket was red after hearing another witness say it was red or after reading this detail in the newspaper. But it may be that the second witness is mistaken or not as certain of events as I suppose.

I think it was Scarlet O'Hara who declared that God was her witness. Scarlet had an omniscient witness. The rest of us are not so fortunate. Let me conclude with an experiment that demonstrates just how fragile eyewitness testimony is. In an experiment conducted by Wright, Loftus and Hall in 2001, students viewed a film of a car accident. They were then asked to imagine and to write down details not shown in the film. These details could involve the arrival of police or of an ambulance. Maybe they involved the arrival of an ambulance chaser. At a later date in the semester the students were asked to recollect the film of the accident. Fifteen percent included the imagined details in their recollections. This is a daunting and scary finding. A sizeable percentage of the participants couldn't distinguish *imagined events* of an accident from the *actual events* of an accident. I hate to think that wrongful convictions have occurred because witnesses imagined details in the course of thinking about a crime. That would be truly criminal.

Thank you.

Tips to Students ~
Ways to Improve Memory While Studying

Study alone in a quiet place. Study at the same time and place everyday. Get into a routine, as if study was a visit to a health club and a physical workout. In fact, studying is a lot like working out. The more you do, the better you get at it. And the easier it gets.

Do not smoke, drink, or eat during the study session. Mimic conditions that will occur in the classroom.

Minimize interruptions and distractions. Turn off your cell phone. Shut the television off. Don't play music.

Try to make the topic concrete and meaningful in terms of what is going on in your life. Hook up what you need to know with what you already know. Create pictures or stories.

Involve all senses in your study. If possible, recite the lesson.

Place the most important topics at the start or at the end of the study session. Study for a quiz last (and then go to sleep).

Do not study similar topics back to back.

Do not cram information. Cramming is an inefficient and stressful way to study. Study in short sessions. Take frequent breaks in which you do not do anything intellectual. After every break review the information you studied before the break.

Work from organized materials. Use the structure the textbook provides or develop your own structure.

Review frequently and test yourself on the material as often as you can. A good way to do this is to use index cards and key words.

Use mnemonics as much as possible—acronyms, rhyming pegs, or the Method of Loci in which you memorize a permanent list of concrete stimuli and attach new information to each of the stimuli in turn. Use whatever mnemonics are available. Better still, make up your own.

LECTURE FOUR ~

Learning

If I ask someone on the subway platform what learning is I'm likely to get a rude reply telling me where I can go and how I can get there. If by some chance I get an educated answer it'll be something like "Learning is getting information." Or "Learning is finding things out." Or "Learning is acquiring knowledge." Or "Learning is acquiring wisdom."

All of these definitions are correct in their ways, but none matches the definition we use in psychology. According to psychologists, *learning is a change in behavior due to practice and experience.*

Like all definitions, this one serves as a springboard and as a frame of reference. It is open to elaboration and to qualification.

Change is what learning is all about. Change is what life is all about. Everyone is looking to get more intelligent, to get leaner, to get richer, and to get in better relationships. Billions are spent annually on books and on programs purporting to improve us in every way possible. No one goes to bed at night and prays, "Dear God, keep me exactly as I am." Instead we pray, "Dear God, make me into a better person." We want new and improved versions of ourselves.

In the psychology of learning change comes about through *practice and experience.* Change comes about in other ways, too. The body matures. Four-year-old children can do something they couldn't do at three. The body grows tired and ill. We fail to catch a ball because we're tired or sick or drunk or hung over. And change comes about through persuasive communication. Politics and propaganda and advertising want to change our behavior through the deliberate presentation of precisely chosen words and images.

You may notice the emphasis in the definition is on *behavior* rather than on cognition or on information or on that elusive thing called "wisdom." Psychology prefers to focus on what people *say and do* rather than on thoughts or ideas. It frequently happens after a quiz that a student says, "I really knew the material, but I bombed out." I don't know what the student knows. I'm not God. I can't peer into the unlit place in the mind where the information hid while the student took the quiz. I can only hold the paper up and look at the score and ponder the shame the student brought on himself and on his family.

The student says, "I flunked, but if you pass me, I'll change the oil in your car." Maybe I'll take the student up on the offer—it is time for an oil change. If the student changes the oil successfully, I'll change the grade and think, "He really knows how to change oil." If the student leaves a puddle of oil in my driveway, I won't change the grade and I'll think, "He really doesn't know how to change oil."

The topic of learning in psychology has always had a pragmatic element. The proof is in the pudding, as they say. Or the proof is in getting a passing score on the quiz. Or the proof is in changing the professor's oil—I should say in changing the oil in the professor's car.

In America the topic of learning in psychology has been closely associated with the behavioral perspective and with behaviorism. This association is not true in Europe and in other places. Both of these perspectives insist on an objective and experimental approach to learning and both shy away from cognitive concepts. Most of the behaviorists can be considered learning psychologists. However, not all psychologists who study learning are behaviorists.

The ability to change due to practice and experience exists throughout the animal kingdom. For all I know it exists in the plant kingdom as well. This ability is brought to its greatest degree in *Homo sapiens*. This ability adds a huge evolutionary advantage and has enabled humans to become the dominant species on the planet. With the possible exception of the box jellyfish, it has enabled us to become the dominant predator. Lower organisms change due to practice and experience. But lower organisms are limited by the instincts or species-specific behavior evolution has endowed them with. They cannot surmount or circumvent species-specific behavior. Humans change due to practice and experience and are not limited by species-specific behavior. What's more, humans change due to the practice and experience of other people.

There's a terrifying documentary they air during pledge week on the educational networks. There's a river someplace in Africa—I'm sure there's more than one river in Africa. This particular river is inhabited by a mine field of crocodiles. A herd of wildebeests has the unfortunate task of having to cross this river. I don't know, maybe they have someplace to go. The first one plunges in and promptly gets eaten. The second one plunges in and gets eaten. The same savage fate happens to the third and to the fourth. Soon, the entire herd plunges in. Most make it—this is what traveling in a herd is meant to accomplish. A lot don't. The river is a bloody mess with wildebeest carcasses floating downstream and crocodiles chomping aggressively. If you're having dinner while you watch this, you probably pass on the cutlets.

Think how humans would behave at the river. The first human plunges in and gets eaten. The second human plunges in and gets eaten. The rest of us aren't plunging in. We start looking for a different place to cross. And we probably put a sign up, "Watch out for crocodiles."

There are two vast traditions in learning psychology. The first tradition is *classical conditioning* that was initially described by Ivan Pavlov in Russia. The second tradition is *operant conditioning* that was initially described by Edward Thorndike in America and was brought to its fullest treatment by B.F. Skinner, the notorious behaviorist. Each of these traditions is tied to experimental procedures and each, as I said, is truly vast in scope, with thousands of published papers and books. The study of classical and operant conditioning is a worldwide endeavor. The study has involved species ranging from protozoa and planaria to ourselves.

In classical conditioning change is brought about by pairing one stimulus with a second stimulus. The second stimulus may be biologically relevant. In operant conditioning change is brought about by manipulating the consequences of a response. I'll describe classical conditioning and then we'll move onto operant conditioning.

Picture this. The time is the dawn of the twentieth century. The place is St. Petersburg, Russia. It's a snowy morning—mornings are often snowy in St. Petersburg. Ivan Pavlov (1849-1936)—the name was correctly spelled "Pawlow," but the "w's" lost a scoop in translation—is a middle-aged man and a famous scientist. He's already won a Nobel Prize for his research on digestion—greater fame is soon to come. He's studying saliva, which is the first step in the digestive process. A dog is behind glass and hooked up to a harness so it can't walk around. Surgery has been done to the dog's snout, so saliva flows into a test tube rather than out the dog's mouth. The test tube allows for the precise measurement of saliva. It's wet and messy work, but this kind of research wins people Nobel Prizes.

Pavlov arrives at the lab. He brushes the snowflakes off the shoulders of his fur coat. He hands the coat to a graduate assistant. He removes his fur hat—a canary flies away. He hands the hat to a graduate assistant. He sits. A graduate assistant slides his boots off and replaces them with slippers. Another graduate assistant hands him a hot toddy in a teacup. I had a hot toddy once—I know its effect. I was in the hills of County Roscommon in the Ould Country. It was an August night, but it was cold and I was shivering. A cousin said to wait a moment. He went inside the cabin and brewed a hot toddy, which is tea braced with whiskey. I took a few sips and I instantly started sweating. He must have gone light with the tea.

So Pavlov starts to sweat. And he gets down to business. He proceeds to the glass. The dog sees Pavlov and starts to salivate. The dog is responding to Pavlov. The dog associates Pavlov with meat. We suspect the dog anticipates meat is on the way. Sometimes I think the dog anticipated taking a bite out of Pavlov. It was this observation of increased saliva that led to classical conditioning. It was a serendipitous observation and it led Pavlov to abandon the study of digestion and to focus on the origin of the response the dog made before it was offered a piece of meat. Pavlov spent the rest of his long life studying what became classical conditioning. He remained an active researcher into his 80s. We might say he was a dogged investigator.

Note the importance of serendipity—penicillin is another example and not unimportant. Pavlov wasn't planning to switch directions in his career and he didn't expect that a squirt of saliva into a test tube would lead to this portion of the learning lecture. I'm sure if I were in that lab and just had a few sips of a hot toddy, a squirt of saliva would lead to nothing. I'd have gotten on with the schedule of experiments for the day, which is a way of saying I'm no Pavlov.

It's not easy to define classical conditioning. I'm going to suggest two orientations by way of a definition. And I'm going to provide the structure of classical conditioning.

The first orientation is *stimulus substitution*. We can consider classical conditioning a kind of stimulus substitution. One stimulus comes to substitute for a second stimulus. The first stimulus is usually considered neutral at the outset. The second stimulus is often, although not always, biologically relevant. To say the same thing from a different perspective, in classical conditioning the organism comes to respond to one stimulus as it does to the other stimulus.

The second orientation involves the process by which a *neutral stimulus acquires meaning*. The neutral stimulus acquires meaning by being paired with a stimulus that already possesses a meaning.

Let's move onto the *structure of classical conditioning*. Classical conditioning begins with a *reflex*. A reflex is defined as *an unlearned response to an unlearned stimulus*. When God and Darwin made us they programmed a number of reflexes in us. Babies are loaded with reflexes. Put a nipple in baby's mouth and baby sucks. No baby has to learn to suck, not even babies from the Chelsea neighborhood. Touch baby on the cheek. Baby turns in the direction she's touched. Place your finger in baby's palm. Baby's fingers close around your finger. Run your finger upward from the baby's heel to the toes. Initially, the toes curl backward. Later, baby's toes curl inward. This reflex is called the Babinsky reflex after the doctor who first described it. Hold baby and pretend to drop baby. Baby's eyes and mouth open. The arms extend forward. The spine stiffens. This is the startle reflex and it's obvious that baby's preparing for a landing. Blow pepper in baby's face. Baby sneezes. But, of course, you don't want to do that. Give baby a spoonful of Gerber's baby food. Baby salivates, just like Pavlov's dog.

Adults have reflexes, too, but the cerebral cortex has grown over the more primitive—dare I say "reflexive?"—parts of the brain. Guys can override the usual response of withdrawal from painful stimuli and keep their hands over candles to impress their dates. I would think chocolates are as impressive, but some guys like to act tough. And we can stifle a sneeze if we're on the lam from the law and hiding in a dusty closet when the G-men knock down the door to the apartment.

One reflex adults can't override is the reflex involving light and the pupils of the eyes. When we go from bright light into darkness, say from the lobby into a dark movie theater, we can't make out any details until the pupils of our eyes dilate and let in whatever light is available. When the movie is over and we return to the lobby, the opposite occurs. We have to shield our eyes from the bright lights until the pupils constrict and reduce the amount of light entering the eyes.

Pavlov was studying the salivary reflex. No dog has to learn to salivate to a piece of meat. Babies don't have to learn this. Adults don't have to learn this. The piece of meat serves as an unlearned stimulus that produces the unlearned response of salivating. Pavlov was a Russian version of a behaviorist and he didn't like the word "learning." It carries too much semantic baggage—remember the beginning of this lecture when we asked undistinguished members of the lumpen class to define learning. And Pavlov engaged in precise experimental manipulations. So he used the terms *unconditioned stimulus* and *unconditioned response* to check the baggage on the experimental voyage. "Unconditioned" is used in the sense that the effect of the stimulus and the occurrence of the response precede any experimental manipulation.

In actuality, Pavlov used the term "unconditional" rather than "unconditioned." The term was wrongly translated from the Russian. You might note that there were problems in translation in scholarly circles in that era.

The terms can be abbreviated, which lessens the strain on the muscles in our writing hands. Unconditioned stimulus can be abbreviated as "US." Unconditioned response can be abbreviated as "UR."

Pavlov needed a neutral stimulus which he could pair with the reflex. He was too important to serve as a stimulus and he might have been a little wobbly from the hot toddy. His graduate assistants were too busy waiting on him to serve as stimuli. So he initially used a metronome, which is a gizmo musicians use to tune instruments—it makes a clicking sound as it goes back and forth repetitively. Nervous people use it to tune themselves. So do bored people. Since many people, myself included, are unfamiliar with a metronome I'll exchange it for the familiar, but actually unused, bell.

So we pair a bell with a piece of meat. Bell-meat. Bell-meat. Bell-meat. A single pairing of bell and meat a day for many days. The dog already knew to salivate to the meat. When we pair the bell with the meat and do this often enough, the dog comes to salivate to the bell as it does to the meat. Maybe not with the same intensity, but it salivates to the bell nevertheless. Bell-meat-saliva. Bell-meat-saliva. Bell-meat-saliva. Bell-saliva.

Let's return to the structure of classical conditioning. We already know that the unconditioned stimulus produces the unconditioned response. We have to add the bell. It starts out neutral but soon becomes a learned stimulus. It produces a learned response. As we know, Pavlov avoided the word "learned." So the bell is the *conditioned stimulus*. The bell produces a *conditioned response*. The term "conditioned" is used in the sense that the effect of the stimulus and the occurrence of the response depends on the experimental manipulation. In a broader sense the effect depends on practice and experience.

These terms can also be abbreviated. Conditioned stimulus can be abbreviated as "CS." Conditioned response can be abbreviated as "CR." The strain on the muscles is further reduced.

In our example the unconditioned stimulus is the meat. The conditioned stimulus is the bell. The unconditioned response is salivation. The conditioned response is also salivation. In many, but not all, examples of classical conditioning the conditioned response is a reduced or less intense version of the unconditioned response.

Classical conditioning is a process that has two mothers. The mothers are *repetition* and *contiguity*. Repetition means exactly that— bell-meat over and over. Contiguity means side by side in space and time. One stimulus side by side with a second stimulus. Bell side by side with meat. There can be no delay between the stimuli. We're talking the order of a second. What if Pavlov rang a bell and stepped out for a second hot toddy? The dog would never associate bell and meat. In addition, the conditioned stimulus must precede the unconditioned stimulus by a second or it must overlap the unconditioned stimulus. The unconditioned stimulus cannot come first. Classical conditioning does not work if it does. If you own a dog, try this. Feed the dog its chow and stand over it ringing a bell as it eats. The dog will ignore the bell and keep eating.

Contiguity and the order of stimuli are easy to remember. In the alphabet the "c" in the term "conditioned stimulus" comes before the "u" in the term "unconditioned stimulus."

Let's look at this example in the context of our attempt to define classical conditioning. The dog treats the bell as equivalent, or roughly equivalent, to the meat. It salivates to both. The bell is in a sense substituting for the meat—it certainly *signals* that the meat is coming.

In terms of acquiring meaning we can ask what a bell means to a dog that never heard one. These dogs were not St. Petersburg street dogs, they were laboratory born and bred. The bell means nothing to such a dog. Pair the bell with meat and the bell means something—meat is on the way.

If we paired the bell with the unconditioned stimulus of electric shock, the bell would mean something different. A different dog stands in a harness so it can't walk around. We ring a bell and a second later we shock the right front paw. The paw withdraws from the pain. Withdrawal is the unconditioned response. Bell-shock-paw goes up. Bell-shock-paw goes up. If we pair bell and shock often enough, the paw will go up as soon as the bell sounds and before the shock turns on. Withdrawal to the bell is the conditioned response. The well-trained dog will likely stand with its paw raised just to be on the safe side and avoid the shock altogether. This process is called *avoidance learning* and it is an important learning process.

Consider the very definition of learning. The dog started out making no response to the bell. Because of practice and experience the dog salivates to the bell. If we want to use cognitive terms, something Pavlov avoided—he's dead so he can't complain—the dog started out not knowing what the bell means. Because of practice or experience, the dog now knows what the bell means.

Let me describe a few examples of classical conditioning involving sounds. Maybe you own a cat. Maybe you've come into some money and splurged and bought an electric can opener. The can opener makes a buzzing sound. The buzzing sound means nothing to a cat that's never heard it before. But if we pair the buzzing sound with the aroma of Nine Lives Chicken, the buzzing sound comes to mean something. Buzzing sound-Nine Lives Chicken. Buzzing sound-Nine Lives Chicken. The cat comes running to the counter. The buzzing sound signals that dinner is coming. The cat is likely thinking, "Humn, humn, good." But we don't know what the cat is thinking. Remember that Pavlov preferred to use objective measures. To be sure there was conditioning, we have to perform surgery on the cat and insert a test tube under the jaw to catch the saliva. We can tease the cat and play with the can opener without opening Nine Lives. The conditioned cat will come running at the sound. We better be careful we don't do this too often. When they get annoyed, cats hiss and go for the eyes.

In this example the buzzing sound is the conditioned stimulus. The smell of chicken wafting through the apartment is the unconditioned stimulus. The saliva we catch in the test tube to the smell of chicken is the unconditioned response. No cat has to learn this, not even cats from Greenwich Village. The saliva we catch to the sound of the can opener is the conditioned response. As with the bell-meat example, the amount of saliva to the sound of the can opener is less than it is to the smell of chicken.

Let me describe another example. In the country of New Jersey there's a fleet of ice cream trucks called Mr. Softee that ride around in summer. The trucks play a distinctive jingle on the loudspeaker. I'm not going to hum the jingle for you, because you'll lose respect for me. Besides, you know the jingle. You know it because you've experienced it. Let's take a child who has never heard the jingle. Maybe the child is a relative from overseas. All right, here comes the sound of the jingle and here comes the truck. The jingle means nothing to the child because the child has never heard it before. We lead the child by the hand and buy him a strawberry ice cream cone with sprinkles. Tomorrow, when the child hears the jingle he'll run to be first on line. He knows what the jingle means. The child is likely thinking, "Humm, humm, good." Like Pavlov, we prefer to use objective measures. We have to perform surgery on the child and insert a test tube under the jaw to catch the saliva.

In this example, the jingle is the conditioned stimulus. The strawberry cone with sprinkles is the unconditioned stimulus. The saliva secreted to the ice cream is the unconditioned response. No child has to learn this, not even a child from across the sea. The saliva secreted to the jingle is the conditioned response.

The sound of the jingle would mean something different if the child received a cone filled not with strawberry ice cream but with worms and maggots under the sprinkles. The meaning of a stimulus depends on what it is paired with—this is called "experience." This is also called "association."

The thought occurs that sounds frequently signal the appearance of food. Bells ring in warehouses. Bells ring in schools. I recollect when I was a cowhand on Antelope Island in the Great Salt Lake in Utah that Ma announced our grub was served by ringing a bell. We immediately raced down the grassless slope to be first at the table. Sometimes Ma rang the bell and didn't serve any grub. She just wanted to see twelve sweaty cowhands charge downhill. No one complained about this. Ma wasn't the kind of woman men complained to. Or about.

The *dependent variable* or test of learning is the conditioned response. Bell-meat-saliva. Bell-meat-saliva. Bell-meat-saliva. Bell—what happens after the bell rings is the dependent variable. If there is saliva to the bell, we have conditioning. If there is no saliva to the bell, there is no conditioning and more pairings have to be performed. Maybe you have a dachshund in your lab. You should have gone with a German shepherd.

The conditioned response *prepares* the organism for the unconditioned stimulus. The paw starts to rise to avoid the shock. The dog's mouth starts to salivate before it gets the meat. Mine does when I approach the bakery. In a sense the conditioned response starts to move forward in time and to precede the unconditioned stimulus. Think about what happens when you start using an alarm clock. The first morning you sleep through the alarm. The second morning the alarm clock wakes you up. You shut the alarm off as it rings. What happens on the third morning? You wake up and shut the alarm off before it rings. The conditioned response of waking up occurs before the unconditioned stimulus of the alarm.

The *key or controlling element* in classical conditioning is the unconditioned stimulus. If it is present, we have conditioning. Consider what would happen if we simply rang a bell without presenting the unconditioned stimulus of meat. Bell-nothing. Bell-nothing. Bell-nothing. Nothing would happen. If we want conditioning to occur, we have to present an unconditioned stimulus every so often.

If the unconditioned stimulus was present and then removed from the situation and no longer presented, we have the process of *extinction* or, as Pavlov preferred, *inhibition*. Our dog is well trained. A bell sounds and it promptly salivates. But the situation has changed. Meat no longer follows the bell. It's no longer bell-meat-saliva. It's bell-nothing. Our dog has to learn this. Bell-nothing. Our dog salivates. Bell-nothing. Our dog continues to salivate. We don't know what the dog is thinking, but it's something like, "What happened to the meat?" If our dog is an anxious breed, it's probably thinking, "What did I do wrong?"

If the bell is no longer followed by the meat, although it once was, the dog eventually stops salivating. Why waste saliva over bells that are never followed by meat?

American psychologists tended to view extinction as a de-conditioning or erasure process. Less and less saliva is produced until the test tube stays dry. Pavlov tended to view extinction as a kind of re-conditioning. First it was bell-meat. Then it was bell-nothing.

Bell-nothing replaces or inhibits bell-meat. The dog learned one association—bell-meat. Now it learns another association—bell-nothing. The new association of bell-nothing blocks the old association of bell-meat-saliva from occurring.

Re-conditioning rather than de-conditioning is supported by the phenomenon of *spontaneous recovery*. We remove the dog from the lab after the salivary conditioned response has been completely inhibited. After a period of time has elapsed we return the dog to the lab, put it back in the harness, and ring a bell—even the folks from Coney Island know what's going to happen. The dog promptly salivates to the bell quite as if it were in the lab and in training all the time. It's easy to re-condition the dog at this point. Of course, if we ring the bell and present no meat, the dog rapidly stops salivating.

Let me describe two additional concepts involving classical conditioning. These concepts are generalization and discrimination. *Generalization is the process in which an organism responds to a range of similar conditioned stimuli. Discrimination is the process in which an organism responds to a specific conditioned stimulus and to no other.* In both phenomena the response involves a conditioned response.

Which process occurs depends on the presence or absence of the unconditioned stimulus. Let's use three stimuli—as experimenters we control the situation. We'll use three bells, each precisely defined in pitch and volume. We have a loud bell, a moderate bell, and a low or soft bell. If we desire to demonstrate generalization we simply follow each bell with meat. Loud bell-meat. Saliva follows. Moderate bell-meat. Saliva follows. Soft bell-meat. You can guess what follows.

The situation with discrimination is more complicated. If we want to demonstrate discrimination we pair the unconditioned stimulus of meat with one bell. Let's say we pair the meat only with the moderate level bell. So, loud bell-nothing. Moderate bell-meat. Soft bell-nothing. Early in the learning process something interesting occurs. The dog spontaneously salivates to all three bells. The loud and the soft bells are not followed by meat, but the dog exhibits generalization and salivates to them because they are bells that sound similar to the moderate level bell.

As the learning process continues the dog stops salivating to the loud bell and to the soft bell. In their cases inhibition occurs. Loud bell-nothing. Soft bell-nothing. This is what the dog is coming to learn. Again, why waste saliva over bells that are never followed by meat?

We have here an important learning principle. The process of learning begins as generalization—if one bell is followed by meat, then all bells are followed by meat. Remember the definition of learning. Practice and experience refine generalization into discrimination. The dog learns which stimulus to respond to, which stimulus not to respond to.

Consider this example. A family trains a dog to go for a walk by rattling its chain. In this family one person walks the dog. Other family members tease the dog by rattling the chain. Initially, the dog comes running to anyone rattling the chain. But with practice and experience generalization becomes discrimination. The dog learns to come to the sound of the chain only if it is rattled by the right person. If anyone else rattles the chain the dog yawns, scratches itself, and goes back to sleep.

Let me give another example how generalization is refined into discrimination. This happened to me recently at the Acme supermarket. I was on line at the checkout. Ahead of me was a young mother with her child in a carriage. I'm guessing the child was two or three years old. I waved to the child. She pointed at me, smiled, and said, "Daddy." I told her, no, I wasn't her daddy and that I didn't have anything to do with her, but I don't think she understood. What occurred was an instance of generalization. The child learned to say, "Daddy" to all tall and good-looking men. In a year's time generalization will be replaced by discrimination and the child will say "Daddy" only to the right man. In a year's time I'll assume my proper role as a "stranger" and I'll be lucky to get a grin in response to my fatherly wave.

A final word about classical conditioning. In a quarter century of teaching general psychology I have never been asked why it's called *classical* conditioning. It's probably a good thing I've never been asked. I don't know the answer. I don't believe anyone knows the answer. There was a man who lived in Seaside Heights, New Jersey, who claimed to know the answer, but he went snorkeling in the Atlantic Ocean one afternoon and never resurfaced. So, everyone is stuck in a lurch when it comes to the word "classical." The best answer appears to involve the early launch date of classical conditioning and the fact that it brought philosophical associationism into the laboratory. Whether that's true or not, only Davy Jones knows.

Let's move onto operant conditioning.

I'm sure something like operant conditioning was practiced throughout human history, recorded and unrecorded. It likely began—rather unsuccessfully, I should say—in the Garden of Eden. Right from our commencement as a species, parents and educators have used rewards and punishments to get people, especially the variety of people called "children," to behave properly. As a topic of research in the institution of psychology operant conditioning began with the experiments of Edward Thorndike (1874–1949). Thorndike studied cats escaping from confining boxes. He called the process "instrumental conditioning" and believed it involved the process of trial and error. When I was in grade school the teachers practiced a variant of instrumental conditioning that involved the process of trial and terror.

Thorndike commenced the study of instrumental conditioning with his 1898 doctoral dissertation at Columbia University. It is surely the most important doctoral dissertation in the history of psychology. When I found out that Thorndike studied, and later taught, at Columbia I wrote then Mayor David Dinkins that New York should name a street after him or at the least one of those tiny corner parks that attract pigeons and derelicts. Most street and park names are pretty obscure. The nearby corner park at West Broadway and Reade St. is named for James Bogardus. It took a Google search to find out that Bogardus was an architect who lived from 1800-1847. I'm sure he was well known in his time, but that time was long ago. Unfortunately, I never got a reply from Mayor Dinkins. I even put a self-addressed stamped envelop for the mayor's convenience—New York was undergoing financial hardship at the time and I thought I'd save them the cost of a stamp. But I got nothing in reply, not so much as a form letter, thanking me for my interest.

Operant conditioning is most closely associated with B.F. Skinner, who is ranked among the most prominent psychologists of all time. Skinner was born in Pennsylvania in 1904 and died as an old gent in 1990. Skinner taught at a number of universities, but he is most associated with Harvard. Skinner was a prominent experimenter and he was, like John Watson, an outspoken advocate for the behavioral—behaviorist—perspective. Skinner worked with pigeons and rats, but he was never shy about generalizing the principles of operant conditioning to human beings. He wanted to design entire cultures based on operant conditioning. In the 1970s communes were established to put his ideas into practice. And he once suggested that we could condition a nation of avid gamblers to such an extent we could replace revenue from taxation with revenue from gambling. That never happened and I think Skinner was a little behind the eight ball with the idea that we could create a nation of gamblers.

Skinner defined an exceedingly useful dependent variable—*rate of response*. Rate of response is a brilliantly simple and applicable dependent variable. It involves counting responses—behaviorists love to count things—and it applies whether we want to increase or decrease the occurrence of a response.

Following up on what Thorndike discovered, Skinner found that he could *change the rate of a response by manipulating the immediate consequences of the response.* The independent variable of the immediate consequences of a response affects the dependent variable of rate of response. To say the same thing without the concepts of variables, the central idea in operant conditioning is that *the immediate consequences of a response affect the rate of the response.*

I suppose there are many kinds of consequences, but in operant conditioning two rather obvious consequences are featured—favorable or desirable consequences and unfavorable or undesirable consequences. *Favorable consequences are called reinforcers. Unfavorable consequences are called punishers.*

Reinforcers increase the rate of a response. The entire process of presenting favorable consequences after a response and increasing the rate of a response is called *reinforcement.*

Punishers decrease the rate of a response. The entire process of presenting unfavorable consequences after a response and decreasing the rate of a response is called *punishment.*

Some reinforcers are biological. In the old days they called biological reinforcers "primary." *Primary reinforcers* include food to a hungry organism, water to a thirsty organism, warmth to a cold organism, and coolness to a hot organism. Some punishers are biological or primary. *Primary punishers* include hunger and thirst and cold and warmth. Primary punishers also include pain—the pain of a broken tooth or a buttock paddled sore.

Other reinforcers are social. In the old days social reinforcers were called "secondary," but this is upside down and inside out when it comes to humans, since social reinforcement for humans is more important than primary reinforcement. *Secondary reinforcers* include praise and prizes and honors and the green paper called "the fabulous moolah."

Winston Churchill once said that no woman can turn down the social reinforcer of a compliment, not the Queen of England, not the charwoman who cleans our fireplaces. I didn't believe the part about the Queen of England until we visited London a few years ago. We were in the Parliament building on a guided tour when, lo and behold, Queen Elizabeth and her entourage got on the elevator we were in. I stared at her. She stared at me. After a few moments of embarrassed silence I bowed and commented, "Your Majesty, your eyes are so blue. They match your gown." Her Majesty blushed and giggled. She didn't say anything, but I knew she was thinking, "Oh, boy." I realized Churchill was correct. The Queen herself couldn't turn down a compliment offered by a commoner.

Queen Elizabeth was not the most famous person a member of my family met. My grandfather met Adolf Hitler. It was in an elevator in the Reichstag building in Berlin. The year was 1936. It was around the time of the Olympics. My grandfather looked at *Der Fuhrer* and *Der Fuhrer* looked at my grandfather. After a few moments my grandfather asked, in German of course, what time it was. Hitler raised his sleeve, looked at his wristwatch, and answered, "Ten after two."

Like reinforcers, punishers can be social. They were called "secondary punishers," but like I said about social reinforcers, this is not right when it comes to people. Social punishers hurt worse than biological punishers. Think of such odious fates as being humiliated or insulted or ostracized. Think of such things as being demoted or fired or fined. Nobody wants to lose their reputations or their money.

Some consequences work by adding something to the situation that was not present until a response occurred. These consequences are called *positive reinforcers* and *positive punishers*. Positive reinforcers add something favorable or desirable to the situation. Positive punishers add something unfavorable or undesirable to the situation.

Some consequences work by removing something from the situation. A response occurs and something that is present is removed. These consequences are called *negative reinforcers* and *negative punishers*. Negative reinforcers remove something unfavorable or undesirable from the situation. Negative punishers remove something favorable or desirable from the situation.

We have four basic situations in operant conditioning. Skinner used the term *contingencies*. They are *positive reinforcement, positive punishment, negative reinforcement,* and *negative punishment.* Positive reinforcement is sometimes called *reward conditioning,* positive punishment is sometimes called *punishment conditioning,* negative reinforcement is sometimes called *relief conditioning,* and negative punishment is sometimes called *penalty conditioning.* It's important to remember that reinforcers, whether positive or negative, *increase the rate of a response* and that punishers, whether positive or negative, *decrease the rate of a response.*

Before we review the basic contingencies I'll like to add two additional points. Reinforcers and punishers *must be defined from the perspective of the person receiving them, not from the perspective of the person giving them.* Every parent has had the experience of believing they punished a child—the child sees the punishment as reinforcement. "Go to your room," the father says and that's precisely what the child wants. Every teacher has had the same experience. The teacher chastises the class clown and thinks the chastisement is punishment—the attention of being chastised is precisely what the class clown wants.

In the same way parents have had the experience of believing they bestowed reinforcement on a child when, in fact, the child sees the reinforcement as punishment. So a parent gives her child money for eating spinach. The child doesn't want the money—if the parent pays for her to eat it, spinach must taste awful. Teachers have had similar experiences. The teacher bestows a star on the child's work. The child couldn't care less.

Finally, reinforcers and punishers must be defined in *the context of ongoing behavior.* I love jelly donuts. I suppose I find them reinforcing. If I haven't eaten a jelly donut in a week, the next one is going to taste deliciously reinforcing. But if I just ate three jelly donuts at a sitting, the fourth is not going to be especially reinforcing. It might actually be punishing. In the same way if I was slapped and spanked a great deal growing up, getting slapped and spanked this afternoon is not going to be especially punishing. I recall what the legendary wrestler Killer Kowalski said about wrestling. Killer was asked if it hurt to wrestle. Killer said wrestling was like hitting ourselves in the heads with hammers. It hurts only when we stop. To a person who is punished all the time, punishment becomes ineffective.

I'll like to describe the four basic contingencies. I'll use two examples. One example involves homework. The other example involves what is colloquially called a "Skinner box." The actual name of the box is *operant conditioning chamber*. I think "Skinner box" is a more colorful term. The box is a glass-enclosed chamber. The chamber has a food dispenser, a tray, and a tiny bar that can be pressed. It also has a grid floor that can be electrified. I would bring one in if I owned one, but I don't. The box is quite expensive and I'm afflicted with the undesirable state of poverty.

Positive reinforcement is the situation in which a response or behavior is immediately followed by favorable or desirable consequences. The rate of the response increases. The reinforcement needs to follow the behavior immediately. It can be biological or social. It must be defined from the perspective of the person or organism receiving it and it must be defined in the ongoing context of behavior.

So we put a slightly hungry lab rat in the Skinner box. The rat has never been there before. It walks around, tries to climb the glass, grooms itself, does it business, and accidentally presses the bar. A pellet of rat food drops into the tray. The rat eats the food and carries on, walking around, trying to climb the glass, grooming itself, and doing its business. The rat accidentally presses the bar and another pellet of rat food drops into the tray. In no time the rat is busy pressing the bar and eating.

Pressing the bar is a response that immediately led to receiving food. Food is a biological reinforcer that increases the rate of bar pressing. The rat entered the Skinner box untrained and not knowing what to do. It left the Skinner box trained and knowing exactly what to do—pressing the bar leads to food. Whatever behavior leads to food increases in rate. Note that reinforcement was not present until the correct response was made.

I should add that the lab rat was a Norwegian rat, otherwise known in Latin as *Rattus norvegicus*. They're quite harmless, unlike the breed I saw last week at the corner of Chambers and West Broadway. An elderly lady was pushing a cart filled with groceries. A huge gray rat rushed from the sewer and grabbed her by the leg. She was thin and frail and unable to fight back. She must have been as shocked as I was. She was pulled into the sewer so quickly, the rat must have greased the grating. There was nothing I could do. By the time I got my cell phone out, she was gone. There wasn't even time to holler for help, that's how fast she disappeared. Only her shopping cart was left on the sidewalk. I felt badly, but I was taken by surprise. I was powerless to intervene and I wasn't about to go in after her.

Let's move onto the homework example. Ma's at the table with her daughter. Pa's in the living room. He's drinking beer and eating pork chops. Ma asks, "What's seven times seven?" The child responds, "Forty nine." Ma reaches over and gives the child a pellet of rat food. No, Ma doesn't do that. Ma reaches over and gives the child a jelly donut. No, Ma doesn't do that. You know what Ma does. Ma showers the child with the social reinforcer of praise. "You're so bright. You're the brightest girl in the apartment building. You're not like that awful girl who lives on the second floor."

Saying "Forty nine" to "What's seven times seven?" is a response that leads to receiving praise. Praise is a social reinforcer that increases the rate of saying "Forty nine" to "What's seven times seven?" The child sat at the table not knowing what the answer was. The child also sat at the table in need of praise—the child is a lot like the Queen of England in this regard. The child left the table trained and knowledgeable. The child now knows what to say when she hears "Seven times seven." Note that the praise was not present until the correct response was spoken.

The second contingency is positive punishment. *Positive punishment is the situation in which a response or behavior is immediately followed by unfavorable or undesirable consequences. The rate of the response decreases.* The punisher needs to follow the behavior immediately. It can be biological or social. It must be defined from the perspective of the person receiving it and it must be defined in the context of ongoing behavior.

So we take another rat and drop it in the Skinner box—actually, we place the rat gently inside the box. The rat has never been in a Skinner box. It walks around, tries to climb the glass, grooms itself, and does its business. And it accidentally presses the bar. This rat has pulled the short straw. Instead of getting a tasty pellet, it gets hot paws. Touching the bar is immediately followed by a jolt of electric shock on the grid of the box. The next time we place the rat inside the box it walks around, tries to climb the glass, grooms itself, does its business, and accidentally presses the bar. Shock promptly follows. Even the people from Todt Hill on Staten Island can see where we're going with this. The rat will not be pressing the bar in the future.

Pressing the bar for this rat is a response that immediately led to receiving shock. Electric shock is a biological punisher that decreases the rate of bar pressing. The rat entered the Skinner box untrained and in no pain. It left the box trained and presumably discomforted. Pressing the bar led to pain. Whatever leads to pain decreases in rate. Note that the punisher was not present until the incorrect response was made.

Let's proceed to the homework example. Ma's at the table with the little one. Pa's in the living room drinking beer and eating pork chops. Ma asks, "What's seven times seven?" The child answers, "Forty eight." Ma rigged the chair the child sits on with a device that gives jolts of electric shock anytime the child answers incorrectly. No, Ma didn't do that. She'd get in trouble with the mayor and the police commissioner. They'll bust open the door and take Ma in handcuffs to the bad mothers' wing of Riker's Island. Ma doesn't administer physical pain, she showers the child with the hard rain of social punishers. She yells at the child, she insults the child, she berates and belittles the child. She makes it plain that the child has disappointed her. "Why can't you get the right answer? Why do you always get it wrong? Why can't you be as bright as that girl who lives on the second floor? She doesn't give her mother any trouble doing homework."

Saying "Forty eight" to "What's seven times seven?" is a response that leads to social punishment. Humiliation and belittlement are social punishers that decrease the rate of saying "Forty eight" to "What's seven times seven?" No child wants to be humiliated. No child wants to be belittled. I'm sure the Queen feels the same—I don't know what would have happened if I said the color of the Queen's eyes didn't match her gown. The child sat at the table in need of praise and was humiliated instead. The child left the table trained and knowledgeable—but wait a moment, the child left the table knowing that seven times seven does not equal forty eight. The child did not necessarily leave the table knowing the correct answer.

Punishment teaches us what *not to say and what not to do*. Punishment does not teach us what to say or do, except by perchance. In the homework example the child gets punished for saying "Forty eight." This doesn't mean "Forty nine" is the next response. The next response could be "Forty six" or "Fifty."

If we want the child—if we want anyone—to make the correct response we have to use reinforcement. Punishing "Forty eight" makes it less likely the child will say "Forty eight." It doesn't make "Forty nine" more likely to occur. If we want "Forty nine" to increase in rate, we need to reinforce it.

Punishment may work to decrease responses, but it is an unpleasant way to do business. It leads to physical pain, as in the case of the rat. It leads to psychological pain, as in the case of the child. People get use to punishment and people learn to get better at hiding responses that lead to punishment. If a child gets punished for using profanity in the home, the child learns not to use swearwords in the living room. But you should hear this child in the playground. He curses so badly, we have to wash our ears out with soap. Finally, punishment complicates situations and makes them aversive. We want the rat to enjoy the Skinner box. And homework should be a situation conducive to learning. We want children to look forward to homework. If we use punishment, the rat fears the Skinner box and the child is motivated to avoid homework. The child knows what's coming—not learning, but yelling and aggravation and humiliation.

Yes, let's set our faces to the bright sun of reinforcement and leave the shadows of punishment behind.

At this point I'll like to stress the concept of *immediacy*. This is a point that is often misunderstood. Operant conditioning works only in the *present tense*. There is no future in operant conditioning. There is no past. Reinforcers and punishers do not work forward in time. They do not work backwards. *They affect the rate of the response that immediately precedes them.* And nothing else. Let me demonstrate this point with two examples. The first involves an attempt to use positive reinforcement. The second involves the problematical use of punishment.

Stan is a buddy of mine. I'm not going to tell you his last name. I don't know who you know. For all I know, you may know Stan. Besides it's not ethical to use people as examples behind their backs. Stan lives in Maryland. Stan has a son, Justin. I'm not going to tell you Justin's last name—it's the same as Stan's. Justin is in his middle twenties and has not graduated from college. Stan very much wants Justin to graduate.

Last year Stan decided to use positive reinforcement to inspire Justin. He paid Justin a hundred dollars for every passing grade he achieved. On December 26th at 2:35 PM Justin handed his transcript to his father. Four passing grades—one A, two B's, and a C+. Stan reached in his wallet and handed Justin four hundred dollar bills. He thought that would inspire Justin to finish school and graduate. It didn't.

Stan asked me what he did wrong. He thought positive reinforcement was a sure-fire technique. I told Stan to give me a hundred dollars and I would explain. Stan reached in his wallet and I explained. Stan thought the reinforcement would extend forward in time and motivate Justin. But positive reinforcement doesn't extend forward. All Stan reinforced was whatever occurred at 2:35 PM on December 26th. Probably, this was Justin extending his hand for the payout. If Stan wants Justin to graduate, he has to reinforce *as they occur* whatever behaviors go into being a first-rate student.

My second example of the principle of immediacy involves punishment. I use to frequent the Paramus Park Mall. Presently, I'm not allowed there—my credit standing is seated. But in the day, I was a regular. One time I noticed a mother on the verge of punishing her son. He looked to be around five or six years. She looked to be around thirty. She was pointing and scolding, "Wait till you get home." I was going to tell her that it doesn't work like that. If she wants to punish the child, she should do so immediately. I didn't say anything—I didn't want to get involved.

Consider the possibilities when they arrive home. Maybe she punishes her son and he remembers what he did. But maybe she punishes him and he doesn't remember what he did. Maybe she forgets to punish him and he remembers what he did. "Boy," he thinks, "I got away with that one." Maybe she punishes him for one thing and he remembers doing something else. Maybe she forgets to punish him and maybe he forgets that he needs to be punished—I suppose it's rather pointless to bring this possibility up. If she wanted to use operant conditioning, she should have punished him on the spot. But that would have been most embarrassing.

I've often wanted to open a store in the Paramus Park Mall where parents could apply the principle of immediacy when they punish their children. They wouldn't have to drive home and punish their children—punishment could be part of the shopping experience. I'd call the store

"Ye Olde Punishment Shop." I'd feature an assortment of rulers, belts, and paddles for purchase in the display case. There would be a Godiva stand and a refrigerated stand for bottled water from Fiji. For a small fee parents can take their misbehaving children inside a booth and chastise them in private. The booths would be soundproof. I think the idea would work. It's operant conditioning in action. The only thing holding me back is poverty.

We've covered positive reinforcement and positive punishment. Let's move onto negative reinforcement and negative punishment.

Negative reinforcement is the situation in which a response or behavior stops an unfavorable or undesirable stimulus or event. The rate of the behavior increases. The unfavorable stimulus can be biological or social. It has to be defined from the perspective of the person receiving the reinforcement and it has to be defined in the context of ongoing behavior. And the cessation of the unfavorable stimulus or event has to be immediate.

Let's return to the Skinner box. We take a new rat that's never had the opportunity. The rat walks about, tries to climb the glass, grooms itself and does its business. Suddenly, shock comes on. The grid is electrified. (We can signal shock is imminent by ringing a bell, but that's not necessary.) The rat squeals and jumps about, hopping from one hot paw to another. It accidentally presses the bar. The moment it does so, shock instantly stops. We can put the rat in the box a second time. It may be a little wary, but it walks about, tries to climb the glass, grooms itself and does its business. Suddenly, shock comes on. The rat squeals and jumps, hopping from one hot paw to another. It accidentally presses the bar. The shock instantly stops. We can be sure that after a few such experiences the rat will be pressing the bar as frequently as the rat that received pellets of food.

Pressing the bar for this rat is a response that immediately led to the cessation of the unfavorable, highly aversive, stimulus of shock. The cessation of shock is a biological reinforcer that increases the rate of bar pressing, which is the response that stopped the shock. The rat entered the Skinner box untrained. After a few difficult trials it is well trained. The training resulted from the rat learning that bar pressing stops shock.

Let's return to the homework example. Ma's in the kitchen teaching the child the multiplication table. Pa's in the living room drinking beer and eating pork chops. Ma electrified the chair the child sits. She turns the shock on. She turns the shock off only when the child says the correct answer. Of course, Ma wouldn't do this. She can get in trouble with the mayor and the police commissioner and get delivered in handcuffs to the bad mothers' wing of Riker's Island.

What Ma might do is to start yelling and humiliating the child. "Come on, come on, why can't you get the right answer? Why can't you be like that bright girl on the second floor? Now, what's seven times seven?" If the child answers "Forty nine" Ma immediately stops yelling. She may even praise the child. If the child doesn't say the right answer, Ma keeps yelling.

"Forty nine" corresponds to bar pressing. Saying "Forty nine" stopped the social punishers of yelling and humiliation. Whatever response stops unfavorable or aversive stimuli increases in rate. Saying "Forty nine" to "What's seven times seven?" increases. The child arrived at the table not knowing the answer to "What's seven times seven?" She left the table knowing the answer. Unlike what occurs with positive reinforcement, a child conditioned by negative reinforcement has to experience the unpleasantness of yelling and humiliation—and she has to make a response to stop the unpleasantness. That's the thing with negative reinforcement—it always starts with something unpleasant or aversive. The unpleasantness goes away, but it occurs nevertheless.

Yelling is a widely used aversive stimulus. When I was in high school I played football. My position was tackling dummy—I made All County second team at that position. The coach was an overweight loudmouth who screamed at us all the time. Can you believe he actually used swearwords? He stopped screaming only when we ran a play to perfection. When I was in the Corps the drill instructor was a tall guy who resembled a street lamp with muscles. Like the football coach, he constantly screamed at us. And he used a lot of four-letter words. Can you believe they use four-letter words in the Corps? He stopped screaming only when we cleaned our weapons correctly.

Let me give three additional examples of negative reinforcement. Two are banal. The third is rather extravagant. They all start with something aversive. Negative reinforcement always starts with something aversive. Positive reinforcement works by producing pleasure. To the contrary, negative reinforcement works by taking away physical or psychological pain.

I have a headache—what could be more aversive? I reach for the yellow pills. The headache worsens. I reach for the red pills. The headache goes away. Next time I feel a headache coming on I avoid the yellow pills and reach for the red pills. I do so because I've learned that the red pills eliminate the misery of a headache.

I once owned a car that made a buzzing noise if I didn't click the seat belt on. Actually, the noise wasn't so much a buzz as a horribly ear-grating, soul-grating, whine. I hated the sound. I clicked the seat belt on as soon as I started the engine in order to limit the duration of the sound. I became so well trained I clicked the seat belt on before I started the engine. I did so because I learned clicking the seat belt on eliminated the horrible whine.

The last example is rather extravagant and easily misunderstood as it involves torture. Negative reinforcement is not torture—I can't emphasize that enough. Negative reinforcement stops torture. In George Orwell's novel *1984* the thought police capture Winston Smith, the book's protagonist. They take him to the Ministry of Love, which is New Speak for the Ministry of Brutality. They want him to love Big Brother. (In actuality, they want Winston to inform on his girlfriend. Loving Big Brother is a bonus.) The procedure involves negative reinforcement. The interrogators place a cage of hungry rats near his face. They're going to open the cage and let the rats nibble on his nose unless he says "I love Big Brother." I don't know about you, but having a cage of hungry rats near my nose is an unfavorable stimulus, if ever I heard one. If I were the novel's protagonist, I'd tell the guards to dispense with the rat cage—I'm madly in love with Big Brother and I'll inform on anyone they ask about. (This is the problem with torture. People will say whatever their captors want in order to terminate the torture.) Saying "I love Big Brother" eliminates the aversive stimulus. Whatever eliminates an aversive stimulus increases in rate. I'm no Winston Smith and neither is he. Smith resists for a while, but the rats are getting hungrier and the experience is repeated nauseously over and over. The novel ends pessimistically with Winston Smith informing on his girlfriend and loving Big Brother.

It's important not to confuse negative reinforcement with positive punishment. They are, in fact, opposites. Positive punishment involves presenting an unfavorable stimulus after a response is made. The rat presses the bar and gets shocked. The child says the wrong answer and gets humiliated. Punishment reduces the rate of a response. We do less of what results in punishment. In negative reinforcement the unfavorable stimulus is present before the response is made. The response removes or eliminates the unfavorable stimulus. Negative reinforcement works by stopping punishment. Negative reinforcement increases the rate of a response. We do more of what eliminates punishment.

Towards the end of his long career B.F Skinner wrote that the best thing he ever did was to define rate of response as the dependent variable. He wrote that the worst thing he ever did was to use the terms "positive" and "negative." He wrote that he should have used the words "type one" and "type two." Students get confused when they hear the term "positive" as in positive punishment. They think people do more of what gets them punished. And students get confused when they hear the term "negative" as in negative reinforcement. They think people do less of what gets them reinforcement. They can't seem to overcome the word "negative" when, in fact, negative reinforcement is a very good thing.

To avoid this confusion, I'll give you question thirteen on the next quiz:

Negative reinforcement:

    a)   increases rate of response
    b)   decreases rate of response
    c)   has no effect on rate of response
    d)   John Fitzgerald Kennedy

I'm sure no one will select choice d). From long years of experience I know a fair number of students will choose b). Students get stuck on the word "negative" rather than on the word "reinforcement." The correct answer, of course, is a).

Before we move onto negative punishment let me mention the obvious fact that in life most situations involve a mixture of reinforcement and punishment. Think of work. Sure, we make loads of money, but there's loads of aggravation as well. Think of school. Sure, it's thrilling to come to campus, but there's loads of aggravation as well. Think of the relationship you're in. Sure, it's wonderful to be with a person, but our significant others cause loads of aggravation as well.

Mark Twain once wrote that some people are thoroughly miserable. Other people are a mix of misery and happiness. But no one is thoroughly happy. If he were a professional psychologist, Twain would have made the same observation about reinforcement and punishment.

Positive reinforcement and negative reinforcement stand in a complimentary relationship when it comes to many behaviors. This is especially true of our vices. People overeat because, gosh darn it, food tastes good. What's more delicious than a mound of spaghetti with two spicy meatballs parked in the sauce? That's positive reinforcement. Some people overeat because they learn that their fears and anxieties dissipate when they eat. Their lives are messed up and out of sorts, their nerves are shot, they're overwhelmed with stress and with worries. They hit the refrigerator and they feel better. The fears and the stresses and the worries go away. That's negative reinforcement—the phrase that's commonly used is "comfort food." The next day they grimace when they stand on the scale, but immediate consequences are more powerful than later consequences. Immediate reinforcements are more powerful than later punishments. We live for the pleasures of the moment. Afterward, we regret what we did, but the future is not here yet.

The same complimentary relationship exists with alcohol. We drink because it's fun to get high. And we drink because of social situations. Think of the role of alcohol in weddings and in funerals. Think of the role of alcohol in dating. What do people say when they meet an attractive person in a bar? A man says, "Can I buy you a drink?" If she declines, he asks, "Can you buy me a drink?" If she declines a second time, he moves on.

Some people have learned to drink to reduce fears and anxieties. Their lives are messed up and out of sorts, their nerves are shot, they're overwhelmed with stress and with worries. They hit the liquor cabinet and they feel better. The fears and the stresses and the worries go away. That's negative reinforcement—I've never heard the phrase, but the term must be "comfort drink." The next day they're hung over, but immediate reinforcements are more powerful than later hangovers.

People who drink too much get physically and psychologically addicted to alcohol. They build up a tolerance to alcohol and require more and more of it to get high and to squelch the fears and the stresses and the anxieties. At this point negative reinforcement replaces positive reinforcement and becomes the dominant process. At this point people do not drink to get high, they drink to avoid the aversive state of not drinking. Without alcohol they get nervous, upset, uneasy, and panicky. They get what is colloquially called "The shakes." They may be on the verge of being physically sick. This is withdrawal from alcohol and it's a miserable experience. Or so I've been told. (The major withdrawal from alcohol is delirium tremens, which is a life-threatening medical emergency.) To reduce "The shakes" people drink. To avoid "The shakes" people drink. This is negative reinforcement and the vice—the vise—tightens.

The same is true of addiction to hard drugs. People use dope to get stoned. This is positive reinforcement. The tolerance builds and people get addicted. Now they have to use dope to avoid the highly aversive experience of withdrawing from dope. They use dope to avoid the noxious state of not using dope.

The same complicated relationship exists with respect to smoking cigarettes. People smoke because nicotine clears the mind and energizes a person. Girls think guys who smoke are from Brooklyn. That's positive reinforcement—smoking provides pleasure and prestige. And then people get addicted. If smokers don't have a cigarette they get nervous, upset, uneasy, and panicky. I suppose this state is the smoker's version of "The shakes." They run outside the building and light up and calm down. That's negative reinforcement. They smoke not to enjoy the experience. They smoke to avoid the noxious state of not smoking.

Negative reinforcement is the cause of all the cigarette butts lying outside the doors of this building.

Negative punishment is the fourth basic operant conditioning situation. *Negative punishment is the situation in which a response or behavior stops favorable or desirable stimuli or events. The response decreases in rate.* A response is made and something favorable is removed from the situation. The favorable stimulus or event may be biological or social and it must be defined from the perspective of the person receiving the punishment. As with all of the operant conditioning situations, the effect—in this case the removal of favorable stimuli—must be defined in the context of ongoing behavior and it must be immediate.

Let's return to the Skinner box. We place a new rat inside the box. The situation is changed from previously. We've placed delicious rat food on the tray. We don't know what the rat is thinking, but it's likely something to the effect, "My rat God, what have I done to deserve this?" We've also rigged the box so that if the rat presses the bar, the food tray tilts and the food goes down a chute. Our rat belongs in the unlucky half of *Rattus norvegicus.* In its excitement at seeing the food, our rat inadvertently pressed the bar. The food disappears and the rat is left scratching its ears.

The rat came into the situation not knowing what to do. It learns, rather promptly I should think, not to press the bar. Pressing the bar results in the elimination of the favorable stimulus of food. The rat learns to avoid pressing the bar.

Let's proceed to the homework example. Ma's in the kitchen with her daughter. The child is learning the multiplication table. Pa's in the living room. He's passed out from all the beer and pork chops he consumed. Ma placed a bowl of delicious rat food on the table for the child to enjoy. No, Ma wouldn't do that. Instead Ma placed a bowl of delicious candy on the table. No, Ma wouldn't do that either. Ma does what a lot of parents do. She showers the child with praise. She keeps the praise gushing so long as the child says the right answer. She stops the praise the instant the child says the wrong answer.

So Ma says, "You're the best and brightest child in the entire class. You're the best and brightest child in this entire building. You're not like that awful girl on the second floor. Now, what's seven times seven?" The child is as unfortunate as our rat—she must belong in the unlucky half of the human species. She answers, "Forty eight." Ma instantly stops gushing and turns away. She may even say, "I don't love you anymore."

The favorable stimulus of praise is stopped when the child says "Forty eight." Presumably, Ma's praise is important to the child. Saying "Forty eight" to "What's seven times seven?" becomes less likely. The rate of the response that resulted in the elimination of praise decreases. The child avoids saying "Forty eight" in the future.

Negative punishment may be a kinder, gentler, type of punishment than positive punishment, but the effect is the same. The rate of response is reduced and we learn what not to say and what not to do. We do not learn what to say and do. The child says "Forty eight" and praise stops flowing. To get it back the child may say "Forty six" or "Fifty." Punishing the wrong response does not necessarily make the right response more likely.

I'll be much obliged if you note that *negative punishment* works by removing favorable stimuli. The favorable stimuli are present in the situation. *Positive punishment* works by adding unfavorable stimuli to the situation. The unfavorable stimuli are not physically present until an incorrect response is made. And note that *negative punishment* is the opposite of *negative reinforcement*. Negative punishment works by removing something favorable that is occurring in the situation. The response decreases in rate. Negative reinforcement works by removing something unfavorable that is occurring in the situation. The response increases in rate.

Negative punishment underlies the practice of "time out," which was widely used in education in former years. I don't believe the practice of time out is as common as it once was. The idea in time out is that paying attention to a child who misbehaves by punishing the child actually reinforces a child. You might remember the basic concept that we have to define reinforcement and punishment from the perspective of the person receiving it. The teacher assumes she's punishing the child. The child eats the punishment up and converts it to the reinforcement of attention. In the situation of time out the child can no longer receive what he or she perceives as positive reinforcement.

In the process of time out children who misbehave do not receive attention. They may be removed from the situation. They may be sent to a time out desk or to a time out room. When I was in grade school we had a "dunce seat." If we misbehaved, we sat on this seat with our nose against the wall and a party hat on our head. In high school we were sent to the football office where we had to sit out the period with the smelly offensive line coach—he wasn't called the "offensive" line coach merely for his skill in training athletes.

We have to be careful with time out and guarantee that children are not misbehaving in order to get out of class. In this case we're sending children to where they want to go—this hardly qualifies as punishment.

Negative punishment underlies the use of fines in the criminal justice system. If we get caught speeding in the country of New Jersey, we'll get a ticket. The ticket costs us money. It may cost us an increase in insurance rates. Presumably, like the rat its food and the child her mother's praise, we want to keep our money. No doubt, it's hard-earned. Parting with it is aversive. We won't speed in the future because exceeding the posted speed results in the loss of money. Speeding reduces in rate—that's the theory.

This example is analogous to what happens in many homes. Teens stay out past curfew. They are "grounded" and can't go out the following night. The car keys are taken away. Presumably, going out and driving are important. They'll come home before curfew the next time. Exceeding the curfew becomes less likely. It reduces in rate—that's the theory.

There's an interesting clash between learning principles and due process in the criminal justice system. Learning psychologists insist that consequences should follow the misbehavior immediately or as close in time as possible. In New Jersey we have a month to pay traffic fines. I get a ticket for speeding on June 1st. I put the check in the mail on June 29th. The fine—losing my hard-earned money—is disconnected from the misbehavior of speeding. Maybe that's why everyone speeds in New Jersey.

A student told me in a previous semester that he was from Mississippi and that they do things differently there. He claimed that if drivers get caught speeding in Mississippi they have to pay the fine on the spot. The trooper must have a cash register in the patrol car. If they can't pay the fine, they have to wait with the sweaty deputy in the courthouse until a relative wires the money. I don't know if what the student said is accurate, but it's a better form of operant conditioning than what we practice in New Jersey since it takes into account the concept of immediacy.

Let me describe two additional examples of changing behavior by using negative punishment. The first involves a clinical case. The second involves professional sports.

The clinical case involves a child who sucked her fingers. This is a bad practice that can lead to infections and to deformed teeth. The parents of this child noticed that she liked a particular television program. They bought a box set of the program. The parents worked the remote. The program was shut off whenever the child sucked her fingers while watching it. A boring travel documentary on the educational channel replaced it. When the child took her fingers out of her mouth, the parents switched back to her favorite program. This was a canny use of operant conditioning. If the child misbehaved by placing her fingers in her mouth, a favorable stimulus—the program—was terminated. This is negative punishment. If the child took her fingers out of her mouth, the favorable stimulus came back on. This is positive reinforcement. We might even say it was negative reinforcement—a boring and presumably aversive program was terminated and replaced by something desirable.

There's a marvelous example of negative punishment in the sport of hockey. If a player commits an infraction on the ice he has to skate to a booth called a "penalty box." He has to stay in the penalty box for whatever length of time the infraction calls for. Leaving the ice, he puts his team in jeopardy, as they play a man short and are outnumbered by the opposition. The concept is that the player will avoid the infraction in the future. To be honest, I'm not sure the concept works, since we're dealing with toothless violent men skating at thirty miles an hour.

I'll like to describe one more principle of operant conditioning. This is *extinction*. We met with extinction in classical conditioning—it was the removal of the unconditioned stimulus from the learning situation. In operant conditioning *extinction is the situation in which reinforcement no longer follows a response although it once did*.

We've seen how in operant conditioning positive reinforcement leads to an increased rate of response. We might predict that removing positive reinforcement results in a decreased rate of response. Why bar press when food no longer follows? Why say "Forty nine" when praise no longer follows? B.F. Skinner (and others) discovered that the situation is a little trickier than that. The trickiness results in extinction being one of the most poorly applied operant conditioning principles.

Skinner discovered that once extinction commences and reinforcement is withdrawn, the rate of response decreases for newly-learned responses and for responses that were always reinforced. The situation is different for well-learned responses and for responses that were inconsistently and unpredictably reinforced. (The latter situation is called a "schedule of reinforcement.") Once extinction commences and reinforcement is withdrawn, *the rate of response temporarily increases for well-learned responses and for responses that were inconsistently and unpredictably reinforced*. The fact that the rate temporarily increases can cause major trouble if the person intending to extinguish a response *gives in* and recommences to reinforce a response. Great care has to be taken with the use of extinction. The person implementing it must stand his or her ground and not give in. Giving in worsens the same behavior the person is trying to stop.

Consider this not uncommon example. A child has made a career of pestering his mother. "Are we there yet?" he asks over and over. "Mommy, are we there yet?" Mommy has heard about extinction and she decides to give it a try. She will not answer. But the pestering is a well-learned, probably a very well-learned response, and one that has led to inconsistent and unpredictable reinforcement. Mommy keeps her lips sealed—not for long. The pestering increases in rate. Mommy resists at first, but after a while she can't take it any longer and she gives in. The alternative is driving the car off the bridge and into the river. "No, you little brat, we are not there yet." Silencing the little brat may provide some relief (negative reinforcement) to Mommy, but it is a major mistake. Mommy has inadvertently reinforced behavior as it worsened. And Mommy has reinforced behavior inconsistently. Poor Mommy—we have to feel sorry for her. The pestering is going to get worse.

Consider this example. Miss Oldfield teaches seventh grade. One of her students—let's call him Roger and he doesn't have a last name—has a well-oiled habit of talking out of turn. Let's be honest. Roger never shuts up. Miss Oldfield has heard about extinction and she's going to give it a try. She's not going to pay attention to Roger. She's not going to answer him. She's not going to chastise him. She's going to ignore him. To her dismay, the chattering increases. Even in a public school teachers can't allow a child to disrupt class continuously. Miss Oldfield has to take control and get Roger to shut up. So she pays attention and answers him, like she use to before she began the process of extinction. This may be negatively reinforcing to her and to the other students in the room, but she's inadvertently and inconsistently reinforced behavior at its worst. Roger's chattering is going to increase.

We can note the difference between behavioral principles honed in the laboratory and behavioral principles applied in what we like to believe is "real life." It's one thing to condition and extinguish responses in the controlled environment of a Skinner box in which a lowly rat bar presses. It's quite another thing to condition and extinguish responses in the contentious environment of a seventh-grade classroom.

Like negative punishment, extinction plays a roll in the educational process of "time out." The teacher once paid attention to the misbehavior and now she no longer does. The reinforcement of attention no longer follows the misbehavior although it once did.

Extinction is frequently confused with negative punishment. They have the same effect—a decrease in rate of response—but they involve different procedures. In extinction the usual reinforcement is not forthcoming. Reinforcement does not follow a response. In negative punishment the favorable stimulus or event—the reinforcement—is present and is removed when an incorrect response is performed. In extinction what use to be the correct response no longer produces favorable stimuli. In negative punishment an incorrect response eliminates favorable stimuli.

Let me close this lecture by giving a personal example of extinction. In the development where we live there's a single mom raising a teenage son. He was a major problem for her. He was a major problem for everyone. One day, I was outside trimming the rose bushes and this single mom stopped by. She said, "You're a psychologist and the rumor is you know everything. What can I do to raise my son so that he grows up to be civil and courteous?" I said, "Give me a hundred dollars." She wrote a check and I explained.

I said that she was probably the kind of mother who pays attention to her son's misbehavior and ignores his civil and courteous behavior. She immediately agreed that was the case. I told her to reverse course and to pay attention to the correct behavior and to ignore the misbehavior.

The following week I was on the lawn trimming what was left of the roses and she stopped by. She was in a distraught state. I thought she wanted a refund. "He's gotten worse!" she said. Actually, she exclaimed it. "Oh," I said, "I forgot to tell you that he's going to get worse before he gets better. Whatever you do, don't give in. Do not, I repeat, absolutely do not give in. His behavior will improve if you do not give in."

I'm happy to report she stood her ground. She didn't give in. Her son has become the model teen in the development. He runs errands for the shut-in's. He carries bundles for the senior citizens. He helps blind people cross the street. When it rains he places his jacket on puddles so ladies don't have to get their high heels wet. He's a great kid and he's my single success story.

Thank you.

Tips to Students ~
Helpful Hints in Studying

I'll like to mention a few ways students can improve their study skills and earn higher grades.

Students should *read the book on a daily basis*—read a few pages daily. Read the book in the same place—a quiet place—at the same time. Studying is like working out at a health club. It becomes habit forming. When students get hooked on studying, they feel guilty on the days they don't study.

Take handwritten notes on what you read. You don't have to rewrite the book. Write what you think are the main ideas and concepts. Write what you think you're going to be tested on. Underlining and using yellow marker are poor ways to study because they are passive. Students wind up underlining everything with the intention of reading the book a second time. Writing slows you down, but it improves the quality of the study, because it makes you think about what it is you're putting on paper.

Repetition is the mother of memory. The more times you review a topic, the more likely you are to remember it at quiz time. *Read the notes you made yesterday before you start today's reading.* You'll be amazed how much you remember when you see it in your own handwriting.

Review the notes you take in class before the next class. You might try reorganizing the notes and putting them into your own words. Many students take solid notes in class and then they never review the notes until the night before the quiz. This is not good practice, since there are often gaps in the notes and phrases that don't make sense. If you review the class notes promptly, you can identify problems and gaps in the continuity.

If you read a paragraph and don't understand it, read it a second time. If you don't understand the paragraph after the second reading, read it a third time. If you still don't understand it, ask me in class or during my office hour. This is the reason I was put on earth—to answer students' questions. By the time I got a celestial appointment all the important jobs were gone. Curing polio, writing *Hamlet*, painting the Sistine Chapel, winning the Super Bowl—these were all taken. That left the task of answering students' questions. I understand it doesn't sound like much, but it's an important job and one I do reasonably well.

LECTURE FIVE ~
The Psychology of Personality

The learning lecture asked us to study what might be called the nitty-gritty of behavior. Humans were construed as functioning conglomerates of responses manipulated by reinforcements and punishments located in environments packed with discrete stimuli. The personality lecture is quite different. It invites us to study the big picture and to construe ourselves as fantastically integrated complexities.

The learning lecture got right down to the business of analyzing behavior. There was little speculation, little reflection—but as you know, the behaviorists were never keen on introspection. Philosophy was for others—for psychologists interested in personality.

Personality psychology asks us to consider fundamental issues about what it means to be human. Personality psychology asks us to consider what makes people similar to one another, what makes people different, and what makes people unique. I'm reminded what the "personologist" Henry Murray once wrote about personality—"Every person is like all other people, like some other people, and like no other person."

Personality psychology asks us to decide—to try to decide—whether biological factors are fundamental or whether social-cultural factors are fundamental. Perhaps it is some combination of biology and culture that makes us who we are.

Personality psychology asks us to consider whether the causal factors in behavior lie in the past or in the future. Do we do the things we do because of what happened in the past? Do we do the things we do because we are striving for some future goal or end state?

Personality psychology asks us to consider whether our behavior is strictly determined. Can we escape the influences of the past? Can we escape the stimuli that bombard us incessantly? Maybe we have free will. Maybe we can choose to do what we want to do. Maybe we can choose to be different and not to repeat the things that got us into trouble.

Personality psychology asks us to consider whether there is stability in our behavior or whether we can change. Are we the same person in our habits and attitudes as we were a year ago? As we were five years ago? As we were ten years ago? Or are we different than who we were at some point in the past? Personality psychology asks whether stability depends on something inherent in personality or on something in the environment. Are we the same person because of fundamentally who and what we are? Or are we the same person because we reside in the same environment? Would we be a different person if our environment changed?

Finally, personality psychology asks us to consider our beliefs about humanity. Do we believe people are basically altruistic and generous and constructive? Or do we believe people are basically self-centered and selfish and destructive?

Personality psychology tries to examine the big picture and to consider themes that have perplexed people from time immemorial. We see the big picture even in the definition of personality—*personality is the stable pattern of emotions, motives, and behaviors that characterize a life.* That's quite a definition. It includes everything but the plumbing.

Before we move onto the two kinds of personality theories we're going to review—we'll get to them shortly, unless something bad happens—it's important to understand that everyone has a personality in the psychological sense. We often use the term personality to describe an eccentric or colorful person. We say to the effect, "What a character!" And we often use the term personality for an outgoing and socially adept person. We say, "He's got personality" or "She's got personality" to describe a likeable and vivacious and enthusiastic person. But dull and boring and uninteresting people have personalities in the psychological sense—I ought to know.

I was once on the elevator on campus with two female students. They were talking about a male student in one of their classes. One student said to the other, "He's really quiet." The other student responded, "He has no personality." I was going to correct them and tell them that quiet people have personalities, but then I would have acknowledged that I was eavesdropping. And that wasn't very polite.

The first type of personality theory I'll like to cover derives from the psychodynamic perspective. The theory is called *psychoanalysis* and was created by Sigmund Freud, one of the scientific great men of the previous century. The second type of personality theory is called *trait psychology*. As you'll see, it's quite different than psychoanalysis. I'll outline three examples of trait theories.

Sigmund Freud was born in 1856 in what is now the Czech Republic. He lived all but the last few years of his life in Vienna, Austria. Freud was middle class and upper-middle class in socioeconomic status. He was Jewish by birth and culture, but he did not practice the faith. He was, in fact, an atheist who believed organized religion was for children.

Freud was very ambitious. He wanted to become famous and make a name for himself in science. Today, people want to become famous in Hollywood or in the music industry. I suppose everyone wants to make a video and put it on You Tube and get their fifteen minutes of fame. In the nineteenth century fame and prestige were found in different avenues, one of which was science.

Freud tried a number of possible scientific avenues to the red carpet—the study of eel testes, a model of neurology, the use of cocaine as an adjunct to eye surgery. Yes, the young Freud used cocaine. He supposedly stopped when a friend botched surgery under its influence. I say "supposedly" since I've always thought the old Freud used cocaine given his phenomenal output as writer, correspondent, and therapist. But I don't know that for a fact.

Eventually, Freud settled on medicine as a career. Ideally, Freud would have obtained a position in a university as a teacher and researcher. But he was Jewish in the capital of anti-Semitism and a university position was out of the question. So Freud hung out the shingle and started to see patients. He wasn't interested in a career stitching wounds and lancing boils. Right from the start, Freud was interested in the mind and in psychological disorders.

We have to remember that in the 1880s there was no psychotherapy in the sense we understand it today. And there were very few theories about the mind outside philosophy. Perhaps I should qualify this and say there were very few empirical theories about the mind. Freud was at the very outset of psychology's existence. He was in the starting gate when the fields of psychology and psychotherapy emerged.

Freud spent the next few years seeing patients and developing his ideas. In 1900 he published his major book, *The Interpretation of Dreams*. In 1900 he could hardly be said to be famous—he boarded the cross-town trolley in Austria and no one recognized him. He had a few devoted fans and followers, two of whom became famous personality theorists in their own right—Alfred Adler and Carl Gustav Jung. By 1910 Freud was so famous he had to rent an auditorium to give lectures and hold discussions. When he crossed town in this time period, he took a cab.

Freud's fame increased over the next decades. He continued to see patients. He continued to write. But his life grew grim in the 1920s and 1930s. He developed cancer of the mouth owing to his excessive cigar smoking. The joke was that he smoked because the cigars kept him awake during dull psychotherapy sessions, but the habit led to a decade of surgery and suffering.

Freud's life also turned grim because the Nazis came to power in Austria and anti-Semitism became the norm. Freud was too famous to kill or imprison, so he was allowed to leave Austria. He was invited to come to America, but he didn't like Americans. He had come to America once in 1909. He visited the country of New York and gave lectures here. He then traveled to Clark University in Massachusetts where he gave a series of lectures. Freud thought Americans were loud and rude people. Like I said, he came to New York and he was an insightful observer of people. If he came to New Jersey, he would have had a different opinion.

In any event, Freud spent the last years of his life in England. He died in 1939.

Psychoanalysis is a big theory—they liked big theories in the nineteenth century. It's a theory of the mind. It's a theory of personality. It's also a clinical theory that addresses the causes and treatments of psychological disorders. I'll like to stress that the theory originated in the treatment of psychologically disordered people. It also originated in Freud's observation of people—and of himself. The theory relies on the case study method exclusively. There are no surveys in psychoanalysis, no correlations, and no experiments. Psychoanalysis exhibits the strengths of the case study method—we get to learn a lot about one person and, by extension, about people in general. Psychoanalysis also exhibits the weaknesses of the case study method.

I'm going to review three topics. These topics are Freud's theory of the mind, his personality theory, and his ideas about anxiety and defense mechanisms. After we review these topics, we'll evaluate Freud's theory and address its current standing in psychology.

Let's get to Freud's *theory of the mind*. Freud divided the mind into three components. The theory is often referred to as the "iceberg theory" of the mind, but I'm going to change the metaphor.

The *conscious mind (consciousness)* contains what we are now—this very moment—thinking. Freud was not involved in memory research, but he supported the conclusions we reached about memory, especially short-term memory. Consciousness is a limited portion of the mind. We can think about one thing at a time. Maybe two things, but not many more.

The conscious mind is like an island—I don't know, it's like Staten Island. It sits atop a vast deep sea, the Hudson River, which is technically a tidal fjord at this latitude. The sea is the *preconscious mind (preconsciousness)*. The preconscious mind contains everything in our minds that is not now conscious, but could become conscious. You're thinking about Freud's theory of the mind and trying to make sense of what I'm saying. I'm going to ask you to stop. Start thinking about your trip home. Okay, stop. Start thinking about yesterday's headline. Okay, stop. Start thinking about your favorite television series. Okay, stop. Start thinking about your first day on campus. Okay, stop. Start thinking about your high school graduation. Okay, stop. We can go on all day fishing in the preconscious sea, but I hope you get my point. The preconscious mind is a vast sea in which float all our accessible memories and thoughts.

If you think about the conscious mind as short-term memory and the preconscious mind as long-term memory you're on the right track. Freud didn't think about the mind in these terms, but he's not here and no one's going to tell him.

The conscious mind is Staten Island—it's always sunny in Staten Island. The preconscious mind is the sea it floats on. Many of the thoughts in the sea come ashore—we can think them. But some of our thoughts have sunk to the muck at the bottom of the sea. They're not coming to the surface, not in the ordinary slurry. There is a third category of mind and that is the *unconscious mind* (*unconsciousness*). There are thoughts in the sea of the preconscious that are inaccessible. We can throw fishing lines out. We can throw nets out. We're not going to haul them in. Not unless we enter psychotherapy.

Think about unconscious thoughts as thoughts that are sealed in casks or in bottles. When I was a kid on the Jersey Shore I use to write nonsensical messages—"Help, I'm stranded." "Help, our motorboat is sinking." "Help, I'm walking a plank." "Help, I've been dropped overboard."—and place the messages in old wine bottles. Of course, I never helped myself to the wine. That was for the older kids. I'd cork the bottles and toss them off the jetty and watch them float away. I don't doubt that some unlucky tourist found one of the bottles and spent the rest of the day wondering if he should go to the Coast Guard station.

Freud's theory of the mind is interesting because it suggests that the conscious mind is a wee small piece of the total mind. This is no insult to the fine people of Staten Island. It's just how things are. If you don't believe me, look at a map. And Freud's theory is interesting because it suggests that there are thoughts circulating in our minds that we are not aware of. The theory suggests there are thoughts and motives that we may not know about. There are aspects of our beings that are separate and not included in awareness. That's rather a scary thought.

I said there may be thoughts in the sea of our beings that we do not know. Freud suggested these thoughts usually pertained to two motives or *wishes*. These wishes involve sex and aggression—usually, they involve sex.

People criticized Freud for being a dirty old man always interested in smutty topics. Freud's rejoinder to this was that he pursued the motives that caused trouble in the lives of his patients. In fact, these motives were responsible for turning ordinary men and women into psychologically disturbed men and women. People don't become psychologically disordered because of their religious creeds or their culinary tastes or their liking for certain types of music and literature. People don't become psychologically disordered because of their political allegiances. People don't become psychologically disordered because of their education or work habits. People become psychologically disordered because of the conflicts they experience over sexual motives and wishes they cannot accept.

It is true that Freud advanced the cause of sexual liberation. His theory was developed in a time of sexual liberation—probably, that was why it caught on so rapidly. If it's any comfort, Freud was a prude in his own life. He believed people should have sex only to procreate. If he stated that today, he'd be laughed out of the auditorium.

The brighter students are wondering how something as obvious as sex and aggression can be unconscious and outside awareness. That's rather an important question. As we might expect, Freud gave an answer. Freud gave an answer to every question, which is one of the reasons why psychoanalysis got into trouble.

So how can something like sex and aggression get bottled and corked in the unconscious mind? Freud's answer is the following—*a weak ego flees the facts and fantasies of sex and aggression that are incompatible with standards of safety and propriety.* The key word in that statement is "weak"—weak means a child's ego, literally. Another key word is "flees"—this refers to the concept of *repression.*

To develop the answer, Freud used a metaphor. I'll use the same metaphor, but I'll jazz it up some. Freud used this metaphor in the lectures he gave at Clark University in 1909. These lectures were published in a slim book called *Five Lectures on Psychoanalysis,* which I recommend as an excellent introduction to psychoanalysis.

Here's the metaphor. This classroom is my mind and the students in the room are my thoughts. I like safe and decorous thoughts. I like the thoughts in my mind to be rated PG-13. But one of the students stands up and, God help us, starts a rant in X-rated terms. I can't allow this. So I throw this thought out of my mind and into the hallway. The thought does not go away. It still exists—the hallway is the unconscious mind. And the thought wants to get back into the classroom. I lock the door to keep it out. I talk louder. And the thought starts to bang on the door. The banging is the symptom involved in a psychological disorder.

There's a catch to this process. If you understand this catch, you can become a psychoanalyst. If you don't understand it, you'll have to find a different profession. The catch is—I have to throw the unruly thought out of my mind without knowing I'm throwing it out. I not only have to forget the thought, I have to forget that I'm forgetting the thought. Because if I know what I'm doing, I'm thinking the same X-rated thought I'm trying to be rid of.

Some years ago I was walking in a park. A little girl of about five or six years rushed by on roller skates. She fell when she passed and skinned her knees. She got on her feet, looked at her bloody knees, and cried with a quavering voice, "I better not think about this." I was going to tell her, "Little girl, it doesn't work like that." But I didn't say anything. I felt sorry for her. By trying not to think about her skinned knees, she was thinking about them. Like that little girl, we can't tell ourselves not to think about something. If we try, it backfires and we think about it more frequently. For Freud, repression was not the same as "suppression." Repression has to happen without conscious planning or control.

For Freud the term "unconscious" has a double meaning. It refers to the thoughts that are outside consciousness—the dangerous and disgusting thoughts that get corked in bottles and tossed in the preconscious sea. The term also refers to the act of repression—to corking the bottles.

There's another catch to this process. Repression occurs in childhood because the child's mind is not as integrated as an adult's mind. We can control our minds and we can think about thinking. Children are less able to control their minds and they are not as competent in evaluating the thinking process. (The term used for this skill is *meta-cognition*. Students engage in meta-cognition when they intentionally utilize the principles of memory to improve retrieval.) Repression occurs as children face the daunting ogres of the *Oedipal complex* and the *Electra complex* in the—with apologies to women—*phallic stage of psychosexual development*, which occurs approximately at four to seven years of age.

Freud believed that during these years little boys fall in love with their mothers and act aggressively toward their fathers. In fact, they want to get rid of their fathers. This is the Oedipal complex named, of course, for the unfortunate Greek of myth and drama. And little girls fall in love with their fathers and want to get rid of their mothers. This is the Electra complex named for another unfortunate Greek.

Freud meant these complexes in a literally sexual sense. What happens to these motives determines what happens later in development. A poet wrote, "The child is father to the man." I think Wordsworth wrote this line—it could have been the guy who hung out in the laundromat.

Whoever wrote it, Freud concurred. "The phallic stage is father to the man." And it is mother to the woman.

Obviously, the child cannot be successful. The parent is too powerful. The punishment is too severe. The motive is too dangerous. The motive is too disgusting. Like many to come, the first love affair ends unfulfilled. The child represses the motive—it's safer that way. The thought wanders the hallway and bangs on doors.

Freud believed that his discovery of the Oedipal and Electra complexes were the greatest in his career. This is proof that a great man can be woefully misguided about his accomplishments. There is no one living who accepts the literal truth of these complexes. But there may be a kernel of truth in the idea that what happens in childhood can affect later development. Children aged four to seven are incredibly intelligent and imaginative creatures. They are curious about everything. "Daddy, how far away is the moon?" Daddy tells the boy. "Daddy, how hot is the sun?" Daddy tells him. "Daddy, when did the dinosaurs die?" Daddy tells him. "Daddy, where do babies come from?" Daddy tells him to shut up.

The ever-curious child may get the idea that sexuality is off limits. Daddy doesn't want to talk about it. Neither does Mommy. They don't look happy. They look annoyed. They look embarrassed. At worst, they openly punish the child. At best, they make it plain that this is a most disagreeable topic. The child shies away from sexuality. He or she may not do so consciously—"I better not ask about that"—but may do so without thinking about shying away from the topic. Sexuality has been corked for the boy and thrown into the tidal fjord. The situation doesn't look promising when the captain of the cheerleading squad makes eyes at him.

At some point the child is going to become pubescent—*genital* in Freud's terms. Right now, puberty is breaking out all over the Bronx, which is why we're safe on Chambers St. at the opposite end of town. Dating becomes important, as does sexuality and all the other motives teens face. Freud believed that personality development was like building a house of several flights. There's going to be trouble on an upper floor if there's a weakness—repression—in a lower floor. If the child repressed too much sexuality—if sexuality became overly dangerous to think about and overly disgusting to consider—the teen is going to face difficulties. Too many important motives are walking the hallway, too many are sealed in bottles drifting in the currents.

Let's move onto Freud's theory of personality. At the origin of the theory lies *conflict*. Freud believed that everyone is in personal conflict within themselves. We are all houses divided against ourselves—some of us are huts, others of us are mansions. Psychologically normal individuals are aware of the conflicts. Often, they are miserable because of their awareness of the conflicts. But they know what is going on. They know their motives. Psychologically disordered individuals are not fully aware of the conflicts. The conflicts float undiscovered in the unconscious sea. Motives lie inside corked bottles. Freudian therapy tries to get these individuals to become aware of the conflict. Through psychotherapy they become aware of the conflict and they become like the rest of us— miserable. At least they are miserable for the right reasons.

Freud had a tripartite view of personality. The original component of personality is called the *id*. This is German for "it." The id is the instinctual part of personality. Included among the instincts are, as you might expect, the instincts for sex and for aggression. The id operates under the *pleasure principle*, which means it wants immediate gratification of the instincts. This may not be how the people in Astoria view pleasure, but for Freud pleasure meant keeping arousal low.

The second component of personality is the *superego*. The superego is the primitive voice of conscience. It's not based on religious or on legal or on cultural grounds. It's based on parental discipline and on the almighty parental word "No."

I experienced a vivid demonstration of the superego some years ago when I was earning extra money baby sitting for my sister's child. Gina was around three or four years of age when the incident occurred. Unlike her uncle, she's a lot older now. Her mother told us not to raid the cookie jar when she went out to run an errand. We would have dinner when she got back. As soon as Gina's mother left, I reached for the cookie jar and said, "She's gone, let's have a cookie." Gina looked at me earnestly and said, "Mommy said 'No.'" I said, "Mommy doesn't have to know." Gina said in a somewhat louder voice, "Mommy said 'No.'" I said, "It'll be our little secret." "No," Gina said. "Just one cookie?" Gina practically screamed in reply, "No! Mommy said 'No!'" Now that was the superego in action if I ever saw it.

The third component of personality is the *ego*. This is the executive part of personality. And it's the socialized part. The ego has to handle the id and the superego. And the ego has to handle reality. The ego operates under the *reality principle*, which means it has to learn to postpone gratification till the right time and place. Consider urination and defecation. These are reflexive actions initially. The baby's bladder empties when full even if the Archbishop is holding him. As the baby grows into a toddler he has to learn to "hold it in," even if it means riding to the next rest stop on the Garden State Parkway. Consider sexuality. Immediate gratification can get you written up as a sex offender. The ego has to channel lust into years of dating and courtship and marriage. And consider aggression. The preschooler wants to take your toy and punch you in the kneecap. The preschooler has to learn to restrain the urge to reach out and hit someone.

The poor ego is assailed on all sides by conflicting motives. The id is like the gas pedal to a car. It wants to be kept to the metal on every road. The superego is like the brake. It wants us to drive in the slow lane. The id is like that little red devil sitting on the ego's left shoulder. "Do it," the id whispers, jabbing the ego with a pitchfork. "Don't hesitate. Take it. Go for it. Make it happen." The superego is like the little blue angel sitting on the ego's right shoulder. "No, don't do it," the superego pleads, thrashing the ego with a harp. "Stop. Pause. Hesitate."

Yes, the ego is assailed by conflicts at every turn. The id wants to date the captain of the cheerleading team. The superego doesn't. And there's a chunk of reality to consider. You've fallen in love with the daughter of the chief of police.

The ego is assailed by conflicts everywhere it goes. The id wants to throw his rival for the hand of the captain of the cheerleading team down a steep flight of stairs. The superego doesn't think that's a good idea. And the cheerleader's brother has a third-degree black belt in jujitsu.

Given all these conflicts, the poor ego does its best to compromise and to get the most benefits amid these costs. The ego wants to date and have a social life and the ego doesn't want to be second best. Maybe it sends roses to the cheerleader and a Bruce Li DVD to her brother. The ego maintains awareness of all these conflicts and solutions. They make the ego confused and frustrated and miserable, but it's when these conflicts slip into unconsciousness that psychological difficulties commence.

Late in his career Freud emphasized the importance of anxiety and *defense mechanisms*, which are *ways the ego can minimize anxiety.*

Anxiety means exactly what you think it means. Anxiety is that feeling of nervousness that drops on us. It's that shuddery feeling of dread and anticipation that something bad is going to happen. It's that feeling of apprehension that wells up inside. It may not be the same and it may not be caused by the same factors, but anxiety feels like fear. We're bothered and we're afraid. We don't feel very good about the situation we're in.

Sometimes the id triggers anxiety by demanding we satisfy instincts promptly. Sometimes the superego triggers anxiety by promising punishment for our deeds. And sometimes reality triggers anxiety—a third-degree black belt in jujitsu doesn't like us dating his sister.

The ego can utilize *defense mechanisms* against these bothersome forces. But there is a catch, a big catch. For defense mechanisms to work they must operate outside awareness. The ego must not know it's using a defense mechanism. This may be difficult to understand, but for Freud much of our mental life goes on outside awareness. Remember that consciousness is a tiny island resting on a tumultuous sea of thoughts and desires.

The primary defense mechanism is *repression* or forgetting—as you recall from the metaphor of this classroom being my mind, repression involves the idea that we forget that we are forgetting.

I'm going to mention three defense mechanisms—regression, projection, and reaction formation. There are many more. After Freud died the study of defense mechanisms became a cottage industry called Ego Psychology. This involved studying how the ego utilized defense mechanisms to handle sexuality and aggression.

Regression is the defense mechanism in which the ego reverts to an earlier stage of development and loses an element of more mature socialization. Think of a preschooler who "regresses" when the parents pay more attention to a newborn sibling. Suddenly, the child starts wetting the bed. Suddenly, the child becomes frightened to sleep alone. Think of what happens after a person experiences a stormy break up in an erotic relationship. The person says, "I'm through dating. I'm never falling in love again. I'm taking up origami."

Projection is the defense mechanism in which we observe our unacceptable motives in other people. Let's say I have a crush on Kip. I can't help myself. If you knew Kip, you'd have a crush on him, too. But this motive is altogether unacceptable. When I grew up in New Jersey guys had crushes on the captain of the cheerleading team and not on her brother. So what happens in projection is the ego turns the motive around. I consciously think that Kip has a crush on me. I can accept that—a lot of people have crushes on me. And I can defend against it.

Consider this example. I am filled with insatiable hatred for Kip. I want to hurt him. I want to throw him down a steep flight of stairs. This motive is altogether unacceptable. I grew up in a Christian home in which I was taught to love and respect people and to extend the Corporal Works of Mercy. So what happens is the ego turns the motive around. I consciously think Kip wants to hurt me and throw me down a steep flight of stairs. I'm innocent. Kip's the guilty party.

I hope you can see that projection, like all defense mechanisms, has to work outside awareness. If I know what I'm defending against—well, it's clearly in my mind and I am full of conflict. Defense mechanisms relieve me of psychological conflict. I don't have crushes on men. I'm not full of violent thoughts.

Many people have referred to projection over the years. Jesus says in Matthew 7:5, "You hypocrite, first take the log out of your own eye, and then you will see clearly to take the speck out of your brother's eye." Mark Twain wrote that everyone ought to be concerned with sin—with someone else's sin. We do seem to see our flaws and foibles in other people. We always seem to be correcting our faults in other people. I suppose it's easier being preoccupied with other people's faults than with our own.

The third defense mechanism I'll like to mention is reaction formation. *Reaction formation is the defense mechanism in which we consciously think and feel differently than how we unconsciously think and feel.* If this sounds odd, remember that there are a lot of processes going on submerged in the preconscious sea. Just because we can't see beyond the euphotic rim doesn't mean there are no creatures skimming the sea bottom—or corked bottles tossing in the current.

Kip's back. So is the crush. The motive remains unacceptable. The ego turns the situation around. I hate Kip, badly. I want to hurt him. I want to throw him down a steep flight of stairs. That's what I feel consciously. But I am unconsciously motivated by quite different motives. The conscious motives keep me around Kip all the time—they disguise quite different motives stirring in the murky depths of the mind.

Think of the most famous conversion in history. Saul of Tarsus hated Christians and pitched stones at them. He was always persecuting them. He was always around them. On the road to Damascus Saul saw the light and became Paul of Tarsus. He became the world's leading Christian. He wanted to convert everyone to the new faith, Jews and Gentiles alike. Saul's hatred of Christians shielded the urge to be one of them.

Yes, hate can shield the bewitchment of love. When I was in college I worked in an office on Pine St. It was an unpleasant work environment. A young man and a young woman were always bickering and squealing to the manager on one another. If one came in five minutes late, the other would tell the manager. If one misfiled a proxy, the other ran to the manager. Like I said, it was an unpleasant place in which to make a part-time buck. I found out subsequently that they married. It makes sense. Their provocative feelings toward one another shielded the attraction they felt.

Love can sometimes keep hate from showing. "Smother love" is the situation in which a parent excessively protects a child and monitors every waking moment. On the surface the parent is being a good caretaker—this is what parents are supposed to do. Under the preconscious surface the parent hates the child and wants to be rid of him or her. But the motive to reject the child is unacceptable. The ego turns this despicable motive around and becomes overly protective.

Let's close with Kip. Consciously, I love and respect him. I want to help him at every turn. I want to do the best I can for him. I want to advance him in every way. Unconsciously, I hate and despise his kind of person. I want to be rid of him. I want to shackle his legs with weights and drop him in the tidal fjord. If I'm aware of these motives, I'm a very mean person indeed. I prefer to think of myself as a shining example of benevolence.

Okay, you're so well grounded in psychoanalysis you could nail a shingle on the mailbox. In this city you wouldn't want for patients. It's come time to evaluate Freud's theory.

There's no question psychoanalysis was one of the most influential psychological theories of the twentieth century. This was especially true in America and in the creative community. Writers and artists loved psychoanalysis. So did actors. The popularity of the theory arose in part from the timing in which it appeared. People were discovering sexuality and aggressiveness—I suppose people always knew about sexuality and aggressiveness, but people were becoming aware of how disruptive these urges can be.

The influence of psychoanalysis has waned considerably in the past forty years. There are very few people left who call themselves "psychoanalysts" or "Freudians." Most of these people live on the Upper West Side of Manhattan. They're aging rapidly. The only way they stay alive is by consuming the blood of nubile psych majors.

The waning of a theory, however sad, is how it should be in science. Theories come and theories go. Mostly, they go. We can hardly call ourselves scientists if we believed Freud got it exactly right a century ago.

The major reason psychoanalysis has joined many other theories in the library where they keep unread books is that it has received little experimental support. Repression, the Oedipal and Electra complexes, his dream theory (which we don't cover)—these fundamental ideas have little experimental support. They may well be wrong. Again, this is how it should be. However brilliant, Freud wrote and theorized and treated patients in the Dark Ages of psychological knowledge. Brain science was in its infancy. So was cognitive science. So was the study of dreams. Freud couldn't be right because he did not have the full—a fuller—picture. His concepts were guesses thrown into the sea of unknowing. They were certainly interesting and creative ideas, but they came back empty of data when they were reeled in on empirical trotlines. All Freud's followers and fans forgot how ignorant they were. Freud himself forgot.

There's another problem with Freud's theories—from the get-go psychoanalysis may not be scientific. It's a requirement of scientific theories that they should be refutable or potentially refutable. This means that, in principle, they should be able to be shown to be wrong. At the least, they should be able to be criticized—that's what empiricism and fallibilism are all about, that theories can be corrected, changed, and discarded. Freud wrote at a time when it was believed a theory should withstand all criticism and explain everything. Freud made it difficult for other researchers to correct, criticize, and refute psychoanalysis. He thought that was a strength of the theory. We now know it was a weakness.

Consider the concept of reaction formation. On the surface reaction formation makes sense. We can come up with many examples. But reaction formation is a difficult concept to test in an objective sense. It may not even be testable. Let's say I develop Professor Ford's Sex Survey. The higher people score on the survey, the more they admit they're interested in sex. But what does a low score mean? A low score may mean a person is really and truly a dud below the belt. A low score may also mean a person is unconsciously defending against raging lust. Owing to the defense mechanisms, hate can be love and love can be hate. Prudery can be prurience and vice versa. As a buddy once observed about conspiracy theories—in conspiracy land everything can be its own opposite. This situation makes it difficult to proceed in an empirical sphere.

Finally, psychoanalysis is subject to the limitations of the case study method. We don't know—ethically, we can't know—what occurred in the therapy sessions that led to the theory. We'd like to pry, but we can't. We have only Freud's side of the story. We like to think he played fair and wrote the truth, but we have to remember that he was using case studies to demonstrate and prove concepts he had fallen in love with.

On the positive side, Freud was the first, or among the first, "scientific" personality theorists. His great influence was in his writing ability and in the fact that he was among the first to objectify personality as a topic worthy of study. He set the table for what was to come. People responded favorably and unfavorably to the concepts he advanced.

Freud was also one of the first to set out a theory that tried to help psychologically disordered people. In the time in which Freud lived there was literally nothing, or next to nothing, that could alleviate mental distress. Freud was bold enough to claim his theory could help troubled individuals. We know now psychoanalysis was pretty useless in helping seriously disordered people, but desperate people were desperate for any help. It was to Freud's credit that he came forward and tried.

The second major category of personality theories I'll like to review is referred to as *trait theories* or as *trait psychology*. This category presents a different way of looking at personality than what we've seen with Freud's psychodynamic approach.

Psychoanalysis took a global view of personality, concentrating on the largest aspects. Trait psychology takes a less global view. Psychoanalysis stressed the developmental aspects of personality. Trait psychology offers an unhistorical and contemporary view of personality and a view not based on a person's development. For trait theorists personality is more like a résumé than like a memoir. For trait theorists personality is more like a photograph than like a home movie. Psychoanalysis studied psychologically disordered individuals. Trait theorists study psychologically normal individuals. The usual samples in research are college students, who are trapped in the pool of course credit. We like to think college students are normal. How normal is a different question.

Psychoanalysis relied on the case study method. Trait psychology relies on the survey method. It has the strengths of survey research— rapid data collection and a less cloudy interpretation of the results. It has the weaknesses of the survey method as well.

There is no founder in trait psychology analogous to Freud in psychoanalysis. Two of the most prominent trait theorists across the years were Gordon Allport (1897-1967) and Henry Murray (1893-1988).

A trait is defined as *a stable element of personality that is inferred from behavior*—and presumably captured in surveys.

So I visit a friend and see a three-year-old child hiding behind his mother. I infer "bashful." Maybe I develop a Survey of Bashfulness that can be used with all mothers and their three year olds. I visit another friend and see another three-year-old child. This child cracks a joke— something about an elephant being in the refrigerator. I infer "humorous." Maybe I develop a Survey of Humor in Preschoolers. I visit another friend and see another three year old. This child makes an intelligent remark—something about why elephants can't fit in refrigerators. I infer "intelligent" and develop a Survey of Intelligence in Preschoolers. I visit another friend and see another three year old. This child throws a brick at my head. I infer "aggressive out-of-control devil." When I get the stitches out, I develop a Survey of Aggression in Preschoolers.

Over the past century there must be ten thousand published studies surveying various traits. This multiplicity results from the ease of administering surveys and finding captive college students in general psychology courses. The usual procedure is to choose a few surveys that can be correlated. Often this is done while working towards a master's or doctor's degree. The overall result of this is harmless, I suppose, other than to the trees that gave their bark to the advancement of knowledge and to the college students who gave up the time they could otherwise have put to goofing off. But I'm too negative. Maybe the students can learn something about themselves as they fill out the surveys.

Don't worry. We're not going to review ten thousand published studies. I'm going to outline three trait theories. These theories are the Big Five, internal and external locus of control, and self-efficacy.

The mountain of traits has been shaved in recent years by the development of the *Big Five* trait theory—this is not an athletic conference. These are five traits that are believed to be general categories that apply to all individuals. The five are identified by surveys. The five are *normally distributed* in the general population. Most people score around the mean or average. Extreme scores occur, but they are not common. And the five are not moral qualities. They are behaviors or descriptions of behavior. Each trait has positive and negative features.

The Big Five are extraversion / introversion, agreeableness, conscientiousness, emotional stability, and openness to experience. I'll briefly describe each of the five.

Extraversion / introversion is among the most famous personality traits. On the surface the trait appears to involve sociability and garrulousness. Extraverts are outgoing and have a lot of friends. Extraverts like to party and socialize. Introverts are loners. They don't have a lot of friends. They frequent libraries. They prefer solitude. These differences may contain a grain of truth, but not for the reasons students think. Extraverts are not more inherently social than introverts. Introverts are not inherently more reserved—many introverts are socially adept, although not especially sociable in the sense of attending parties and mixing casually with people.

The decisive difference between the two types is not sociability. Carl Gustav Jung (1875-1961), one of psychology's great men, published a book called *Psychological Types* in 1921 in which he suggested the defining feature of extraversion / introversion is *the preoccupation individuals have with their thought processes and fantasy lives*. Introverts are highly preoccupied with their thoughts and with their fantasies. They find external events, including people, distracting and intrusive. Dealing with the external world reduces the time introverts can spend with their inner worlds. Extraverts are less preoccupied with their thoughts and fantasies. They don't find people distracting because there's less to fascinate them in the private worlds in their minds.

Another view of extraversion / introversion was developed by Hans Eysenck (1916-1997), a British psychologist. Eysenck suggested that *introverts are more strongly aroused psychologically than extraverts.* Introverts have a more highly aroused cerebral cortex and sensory system. They are highly reactive and experience events more intensely. They seek to reduce stimulation and to keep excitation low. This reduction in stimuli may mean avoiding parties and boisterous friendships. Extraverts have a less aroused cerebral cortex and sensory system. They are less reactive and prefer to increase arousal. Noise doesn't bother them. Neither do rowdy events. The introverts are standing on the shore—probably, they want to be somewhere else. The extraverts are in the swim of things. They're happy when the beach is jammed.

It is possible to assess which type a person is by the use of self-report questionnaires. There are many surveys assessing extraversion and introversion. A cottage industry has grown up assessing Jung's model of psychological types. This industry uses a questionnaire called the Myers-Briggs Type Indicator. But we don't need to mass produce surveys on the photocopier to find out if we're introverted or extraverted. All we need is a lemon. Afterward we can make lemonade.

The lemon test of extraversion / introversion is simplicity itself. Slice a lemon in two and suck on one of the slices. If you produce an overflow of saliva, you're likely an introvert. If you produce an ordinary amount of saliva, you're likely an extravert. Remember that introverts experience events more intensely. This includes sucking on lemon slices.

Probably, there's an even simpler test. If the mere thought of sucking on a lemon made you shiver, you're an introvert.

And there's another simple test of introversion. If anyone has ever said to you, "You're too quiet," or "You should speak up more," you're likely an introvert.

As with every one of the Big Five, extraversion / introversion is distributed normally. Most people score average on self-report indicators. Extreme scores occur, but are statistically rare. As with every one of the Big Five, there are situational factors that need to be taken into account. There are situations in which a person behaves in an extraverted manner and there are different situations in which the same person behaves in an introverted manner. I can think of a situation in which an extravert analyzes by introspection some interpersonal problem—why did she do that? Why did he do that? And I can think of a situation in which an introverted person behaves in a highly social manner with a friend.

That said, introverts have a tough time. America is home of the brave and of the extraverted. We're a loud, noisy, brash society. We talk all the time. We never stop talking. The ideal we have is that of the salesperson. Another ideal is that of the celebrity. We want to be liked. We want to be likeable. We want to be forceful. We want to be outgoing. We want to be the center of attention. We want to be on all the social media. All this is well and good, but there is another side and that's the private place inhabited by introverts. That private place is crucial to creativity. Talkative people are rated as better-looking, smarter, more interesting, and more desirable as a friend. But to be creative involves reflection and introspection and solitude. And these things depend on introversion.

Agreeableness involves our attitudes toward other people. Individuals scoring high on questionnaires assessing agreeableness cooperate with people, are trustful, and believe people are trustworthy. Individuals scoring low on agreeableness tend not to cooperate with people, tend not to be trustful and tend to be suspicious of people.

Conscientiousness involves the extent to which people are organized and persistent. Individuals scoring high on questionnaires assessing conscientiousness tend to be self-disciplined and to prefer to stay on schedule. They're the kind of people who arrive extra early at the airport to be sure they make the flight. They're the kind of people who arrive extra early at a dinner engagement and wait patiently in their cars to guarantee they ring the doorbell on schedule. Individuals scoring low on this trait tend to be less disciplined and to ignore schedules. They're the kind of people who arrive in the nick of time at the airport and who arrive fashionably late at a dinner engagement.

Individuals scoring high in the trait of conscientiousness are the kind of people who use a day planner. I'm reminded of an incident a few semesters ago. I'm usually the last person to leave the room—this would not be true if we were holding class on the *Titanic*. On my way out of the classroom I noticed a student had left her notebook behind—it couldn't have been she was in a rush to leave. Ever the diligent teacher, I took the notebook with me and gave it back the following week. I tried not to, but I couldn't help myself. I was tickled by curiosity over the kind of notes she kept. Just what was she writing in class? Not a whole lot, it turned out. Her notes were skimpy. I didn't think she'd do well on the next quiz. Anyway, to return to the point of the trait of conscientiousness, her schedule was at the back of the notebook. On Tuesday she had Spanish at ten AM, chemistry at noon, gym at three, and supper at six. At nine PM she wrote the word "Fun." Now she's clearly a conscientious person to schedule fun in her daily routine. I'm not sure how much fun a person can have if she has to remind herself to have some. On the other hand, maybe this student has a lot of fun on Tuesday nights. I remember a wise piece of advice given me by the most socially adept person I ever knew—this was not a psychoanalyst, but a bartender. "The key to life," Martha said, "is to plan to be spontaneous."

When I returned the notebook, this student asked if I had looked inside. "You didn't look inside my notebook, did you, professor?" "Of course not," I answered. "What kind of person do you think I am?"

The fourth trait in the Big Five is *emotional stability*. Individuals scoring high on the trait of emotional stability express emotions freely and deeply. They are emotionally labile and changeable. This includes the expression both of positive emotions such as happiness and negative emotions such as anger. These individuals tend to be excitable and high strung. They do not handle pressure well. Individuals scoring low on this trait tend to be emotionally constrictive. They do not express strong emotion. They are unexcitable. Pressure doesn't bother them. Nothing sets them off—if there were such a phrase, they would be described as "low strung."

When it comes to excitable individuals I'm reminded of a lady I once saw at the bakery in Macy's. She was crying and carrying on something awful over the fact that they had run out of prune Danish. When it comes to phlegmatic individuals I'm reminded of my cousin Hector, who could never be said to be emotionally excitable. When we visited the Grand Canyon Hector looked bored. He was yawning and playing with a yo-yo while the rest of us were jumping in excitement over the majestic scenery.

The fifth trait of the Big Five is *openness to experience*. Individuals scoring high on questionnaires assessing openness to experience tend to exhibit curiosity about things, especially new and unconventional things. They tend to exhibit a broad range of interests and to be imaginative. They tend to be on the cutting edge and to like the new and the untried. They are independent of the popular culture and of the majority opinion. Individuals scoring low tend to be practical and realistic. They tend to be conventional and to be mainstream in their preferences. They tend to focus on a few well-tried topics rather than on a range of topics. They tend to go along with the majority and to relish the popular tastes. They are fully enmeshed in the popular culture.

Individuals scoring high on openness to experience prefer the avant-garde in movies and in books. They watch and read whatever interests them, whether or not it's popular. In fact, they prefer the obscure and the unique. They tend to take vacations in obscure places the rest of us never heard of. Individuals scoring low on openness to experience prefer blockbuster movies and bestsellers in their entertainment choices. They watch and read what everyone is watching and reading. When they go on vacation it's usually to Orlando in Florida.

An important trait of personality was advanced by Julian Rotter who taught in Connecticut for many years. This is the trait of *locus of control*, which is defined as *the extent to which people believe they control what happens to them*. Rotter identified two orientations when it comes to the belief that we control our destinies.

People who express an *internal locus of control* believe they control their destinies and that they are responsible for what happens to them. They believe they control events. People who express an *external locus of control* believe, to the contrary, that they do not control their destinies and that they are not responsible for what happens to them. Events control them rather than the other way around.

People who demonstrate internal locus of control believe they are masters of their fates and captains of their destinies. Success and failure are in their hands. It's up to them—it's all up to them. People who demonstrate external locus of control believe they are down in the poop deck and rowing. The captains who guide their destinies are somewhere else—let's hope they're on the bridge and sober. They believe that success or failure is not up to them. It's up to fate or to luck or to their genetic heritage or to God or to the Dark Lords who run things from behind the cosmic curtains.

Consider performance in school. Internally-oriented students believe they can get high grades if they prepare and set their minds to completing the coursework. Externally-oriented students do not express this belief in full. They believe a lot depends on getting an easy teacher or an easy textbook. Consider a job interview. Internally-oriented people believe their chances of getting hired improve if they dress properly and practice interviewing techniques and research the company to find impressive questions to ask the interviewer. Externally-oriented people believe that getting a job depends on luck or on God's grace or on being interviewed at the right moment. And consider health issues. Internally-oriented people believe good health is a matter of choice and preparation. They stop smoking, they stop drinking, they lose weight, and they work out. Externally-oriented people believe we can live healthy and work out all we want, but if we step in front of a bus we're going to the Pearly Gates no matter how much time we spent jogging uphill on a treadmill.

Correlational studies indicate that internally-oriented people do, in fact, get higher grades and show more competence and effectiveness. Internally-oriented people are less likely to conform to popular culture and they are less susceptible to influence by others. They like to be their own man. Or their own woman.

Lest we think that it's all peaches and cream for internally-oriented people, consider what happens when they fail. In the same way that they take credit for their successes, they take credit for their failures. They get a low grade on a quiz. They can't blame the quiz, they can't blame the teacher. They tell themselves, "Study harder," "Prepare better," "Goof off less." They get rejected in the job interview. They can't blame the recruiter. They tell themselves, "I should have prepared better," "I should have been more upbeat," "I should have used a more expensive cologne."

There are wide individual differences with locus of control. High scores on surveys occur, but they are rare. As with the Big Five, most people score around the average, being moderately internal and moderately external. And there are individual differences in the kinds of situations people believe they are masters of. Some people may feel internally oriented in intellectual endeavors and externally oriented in social endeavors. For want of a better term we can call these people "nerds." And the opposite is true. There are people who are externally oriented in intellectual endeavors and internally oriented in social endeavors. There must be a word for this kind of person, but I don't know what it is. Maybe we can call them "anti-nerds."

What turns a person in the internal direction? Rotter believed it was consistent parental behavior and access to social power and to material resources. If a person's parents reinforce and encourage active striving—if they reinforce studying and job preparation and clean living—the child grows up with the sense that he or she can compete and achieve. It becomes easier to exhibit an internal locus if a child learns how to behave socially—"how to win friends and influence people," to use a cliché. And it becomes easier if the child has material resources to compete. Material resources include access to information, to good clothing, and to better brands of cologne.

The third example of a trait I'll like to describe is *self-efficacy* or *competence.* Many years ago a psychodynamic psychologist named Robert White suggested that our view of our competence in particular situations was an important element of our self-esteem and of our success. Years later an important psychologist named Albert Bandura revived White's concept as *self-efficacy,* which is rather a sterling word.

Bandura was born in Canada, which we shouldn't hold against him. You'll study Bandura's research on observational learning if you take the course on child psychology. You'll study his views on personality if you take the personality course. And you'll study his views on learning if you take the learning course. As you can note, Bandura made a big splash in the pool of psychology.

Self-efficacy is our belief that we can perform successfully in a particular situation. Do we see ourselves acting successfully in a job interview? Do we see ourselves acting successfully on the athletic field? Self-efficacy orients our personalities and our behavior. If we believe we can act successfully, our thoughts and behaviors shift in one direction. If we believe we cannot act successfully in a particular situation, our thoughts and behaviors shift in a different direction. If we see ourselves as efficacious—there's another sterling word—we are not conflicted and we can move promptly toward our goals. If we don't see ourselves as efficacious—if we don't see ourselves as competent—we are conflicted. We want to move toward our goals, but we're not sure how we're doing and we question our performance. Questioning performance while it occurs is a way to court failure.

Consider going for a job interview. People who see themselves as efficacious aren't troubled by doubts or second thoughts. They proceed with the interview with no cognitive sidetracks. They can stay on the main road. They look and sound confident. They give the appearance of success. People who don't see themselves as efficacious present a different picture. They doubt themselves. They have second thoughts. They're always on a cognitive sidetrack asking themselves how they're doing. Probably, the answer is not positive. They don't present a picture of success. They look insecure. They look hesitant. They look like they're preoccupied—and they are preoccupied with the insistent motive of not messing up the interview. Of course, they promptly mess up.

Consider athletics. I recall going to many Little League baseball games. I observed the trait of self-efficacy in the body language of the players. The players who wanted to be on the field acted assertively. The players who didn't see themselves as efficacious acted differently. They looked like they wanted to be on the bench rather than on the field. If they were on the field, they were in right field, which is where coaches put less competent players. (Most batters are right handed and tend to hit the ball to left field.) I knew what they were thinking. "Please, God, don't let him hit it to me." And I knew what was going to happen. God takes a breather from the important work and directs a right-handed batter to hit a line drive directly at the startle on the face of the right fielder. "Here it comes, oh no!" The right fielder was so busy trying to avoid dropping the ball he promptly dropped the ball. He cost his team the game. His fellow players hate him. The coach hates him. The fans hate him. Even his parents hate him. Maybe his parents don't hate him—they're just ashamed of him.

When people do not feel they will succeed, they may give up and not make the effort. "Why bother?" they ask. "If they hit it to me, I'll only drop the ball." And such people may engage in self-defeating behaviors. They may come to sabotage themselves. They may procrastinate. They may not prepare. They may take on too many tasks. They may use alcohol. They may not get enough sleep.

The origin of self-efficacy lies in the history of successes and failures. If we experience success in particular situations, say socially or athletically, then we may expect to succeed in the next situation. If we come from a history of failures, then we may expect to fail in the next situation. There are many reasons people fail. They may be poorly trained. They may face complex situations—the human resources interviewer may be having a bad morning and the ball may hit a pebble as it heads toward right field. They may be unlucky. They may be told that they are failures. They may be forced to do what they don't want to do. They may be intrinsically incompetent. As General

Burkhalter said of Colonel Klink in the *Hogan's Heroes* television series, "Now, there's Colonel Klink. He could have been great, but he wasn't very good."

Self-efficacy plays a role in the privacy of our personalities and it plays an important role in interpersonal behavior. I'll like to illustrate this with a story. Two men were competing for the hand of a young lady. In those days men had to get the approval of the young lady's father to court her. I don't think men have to do that anymore. One of the suitors got the idea to take the young lady and her father on a one horse open sleigh ride up the Boston Post Road to a Chinese restaurant. He arranged for the horse's harness to come loose. He promptly jumped out of the sleigh and tightened the harness and on the way they went. He had lo mein, the father had a combination platter, and the young lady had egg drop soup and a salad. She was watching her weight.

When the second suitor heard what happened he arranged to take the young lady and her father on a one horse open sleigh ride up the Boston Post Road to an Italian restaurant. The harness loosened again. The father waited, but the young man didn't stir. "Aren't you going to tighten it?" the father asked. "I don't know how," the man replied. "Do you?" The father growled, jumped out of the sleigh, and tore his jacket off. "Come here," he instructed, "and watch what I do." Once the father tightened the harness, they proceeded to the restaurant. The young man had lasagna, the father had linguini with red sauce, and the young lady had a salad. She was still watching her weight.

Which of the young men got the hand of the daughter in holy matrimony?

You would be right if you said the second young man got the daughter's hand—and the rest of her. You're right to think he showed he was incompetent. But notice what he did. He made the father feel competent. He made the father look more competent than he was.

There's a real interpersonal trick here. No one likes a smart-aleck. No one likes a know-it-all. No one likes a pompous person who lords over others. To the contrary, we like it when we appear to be a little brighter and a little more competent than the other person. We like it when we appear to know more than the other person. We like it when we appear better than the other person. And we like the other person who allows us to look more competent.

Consider an example from work. Your boss gives you a project involving Excel. Maybe you have to do a vertical lookup between spreadsheets. But you don't know how. You can spend all afternoon perusing manuals, but there's an easier way. You can go in and say to the boss, "I'm a little confused. Maybe you can help. Everyone says you're the company's leading expert on Excel. Maybe you can give me a few pointers, if you have the time."

He's just been called an "expert." And not just an expert, but "the company's leading expert." How can he turn you down? He's been told he's more competent than you. And you've just admitted you don't know as much as he does. Chances are he'll give you more than a few pointers. He'll likely do the vertical lookup for you.

Back in the day when I was reading things, I use to write authors of psychology articles for reprints. Psychological journals usually listed the author's affiliation and address. And the journals usually supplied the author with a number of complimentary reprints. For example, I'd read an article on anxiety and I'd write the author for a reprint. "Dear Prof. So-and-so, I just read your article on anxiety. I'm a graduate student who's considering a research project on anxiety. I found your article invaluable. It's one of the best articles I've read on the topic. You're obviously a leading expert in the field. Please send me a copy so I can study the article in more detail."

It never failed that I got a copy of the article—and complimentary copies of everything the author ever wrote.

That's the trick in getting people to like you and to do things for you. Get them to feel they're more competent than you. Get them to feel they're more important. Get them to feel they're better. Get them to feel self-efficacious. The secret to getting the boss to do vertical lookups for you is to get him to think he's better than you and knows more than you. And the secret in doing research is to find the person who has and flatter him or her. In the old days researchers use to wait by the mailbox. Today, they're waiting by the e-mailbox. They keep checking, but no one asks for them to impart their special knowledge. "Why, oh why, doesn't somebody ask me a question?" They don't know it, but this is their lucky day. You've just powered up the laptop.

Make the researchers feel like experts. Make them think you're a clueless clod in need of their guidance. Whether in business or in academia, it never hurts to appear less bright than you are.

We can now evaluate trait theories of personality. On the positive side trait theories have led to an enormous amount of research and to the development of many self-report surveys.

On the negative side trait theories are descriptive and correlational. They tell us what characteristics go with what other characteristics. They do not tell us what causes the correlations. And trait theories suffer all the problems of survey research. They are affected by issues of response bias, social desirability, and the wording of questions. And scores on surveys may be poorly related to actual behavior. People do not always do the things they say they do.

There is another danger in survey research. In 1949 a psychologist named Betram Forer coined the term *Barnum effect* to describe the situation in which people endorse vague and positive descriptions of themselves whether or not these descriptions are accurate. Barnum was, of course, the showman whose circus "has something in it for everyone."

I use to demonstrate the Barnum effect in class. I distributed a professional-looking handout called the "Hardy Personality Questionnaire." It consisted of fifty true / false items such as "I like the color blue more than the color red," "I do my best work in the morning," and "I could become a vegetarian if I had to." Each questionnaire was coded with a letter-number combination—R32, for example—"For reasons of confidentiality."

A few weeks later I gave the results of the survey to the students. The results were coded with the same letter-number combination. I urged the students not to share the information. "The results are confidential," I said. In fact, the results consisted of vague and flattering statements. "You are future oriented and you like to reminisce about the past." "You are somewhat rebellious and you have a deep respect for tradition." "You alternate between imaginative thinking and realistic thinking." "You are a socially outgoing person who likes solitude." "You like innovation and you are devoted to traditional ways."

Notice that it is nearly impossible to disagree or to contradict these statements. They are vague and flattering. It would be a different case if the statements were vague and insulting. "You know a lot of people and none of them are your friends." "You are rigid in your thinking and rarely show creativity." "You are set in your ways and show a need for approval." "You could have been great, but you aren't very good." No one would agree with these statements. But when it comes to positive statements, how can we disagree?

As a final step in the classroom procedure I ask the students to raise their hands if they think the statements describe their personalities. Nearly everyone in the class raises their hands. Of course, the procedure is a trick. Everyone received the same set of statements.

The Barnum effect demonstrates that people want to accept what we say about them. People want to believe, especially if the information is coming from an official source, like a psychologist. People take this information—if it's positive—and see how it fits. People will bend and twist and turn the information inside out to see how it applies to them. People will not consider that the information does not apply. Of course, if the information is negative, they won't believe a word.

The Barnum effect demonstrates the importance of keeping a critical attitude. Sure, we like to hear that we're imaginative and rebellious and socially adept, but we should inquire how the information was derived and what the standards of research are. Not a single person in the class asked how the scores were obtained. Everyone was too busy fitting the conclusions to their frames of personality. I should say to their ever-pliable frames of personality.

Thank you.

TIPS TO STUDENTS ~
Helpful Hints in
Reading Textbooks

Preview each chapter by reading section headings, picture captions, and any graphs or figures.

Read the chapter Summary before you read the chapter.

If the chapter has a list of terms, list each term on a piece of paper or on an index card. Write the definitions and any examples as you read.

If the chapter has a list of essay questions, write each question on a piece of paper. Try to answer the question with the notes you make as you read the chapter. If the chapter does not have a list of questions, develop your own based on the preview and Summary. *What do you want to know based on what you read? What material is meaningful in your life?*

If the chapter has a list of multiple-choice questions, answer them. They are likely to be similar and to cover the same material as will appear on quizzes.

Read a few pages on a daily basis.

Take handwritten notes on what you read. Do not underline or use a black or yellow marker.

Before you begin your daily reading, review the handwritten notes you made the day before. Try to develop continuity in your note taking.

If you read a word you don't understand, look it up in the Glossary at the end of the chapter (or at the end of the book). If the book doesn't have a Glossary, use a dictionary or ask about the word in class.

If you don't understand a paragraph, read it a second time. If you don't understand the paragraph, read it a third time. If you still don't understand, bookmark the page and ask about it in class.

To review for a quiz, review your handwritten notes, your list of definitions, and your answers to all chapter questions. Check to see that you've received answers to the questions you may have had about difficult material. You can be sure the content of unanswered questions will appear on the quiz.

LECTURE SIX ~
Brain and Behavior

I'll like to start this lecture by waxing philosophical. Or, as it will be a few brief comments, the phrase might better be "waning philosophical."

I think it is an astounding observation that a three pound organ consisting of cells and water and blood and goo and gore has become aware of the world and, what is more astounding, that it has become aware of itself. The liver isn't aware of the world or of itself. The heart isn't aware. The stomach isn't aware. None of the organs are self-aware. Only the brain is.

I suppose every organism is aware of the world to some degree. The Venus Fly Trap "knows" when to close and what to consume. A jellyfish "knows" when a meal floats nearby. An elephant "knows" where the water hole is in drought season. A crocodile "knows" to lie in wait for a wildebeest to take a drink in the river. Like these organisms, the human brain knows where to find food. In the old days people had to hunt or fish or farm and I don't think I would have been good at any of those professions. Nowadays, we drive to the supermarket and I'm very proficient at doing that. Unlike other organisms, the human brain has discovered, or is in the process of discovering, the physical nature of reality. We know what matter is and what DNA is. We know there are stars out there. We know what's inside the atom. The human brain has discovered so many facts it is tampering with physical reality and with evolution.

This organ of flesh and blood resides in a being that lives for sixty or seventy years. Yet the brain has enabled this being to comprehend the origin of the universe billions of years ago. And the brain has enabled this being to live the entire existence of its species. Because of this organ we don't live sixty or seventy years. We live for billions of years.

The fact that the brain is aware of itself is a strange and fascinating thing. The organ being studied is the same organ doing the studying. This is such a unique fact, it might be useful to stand back and take a breath. I don't know exactly how, but the fact that the brain studies itself is an interesting challenge to philosophy.

The brain stands in a peculiar relationship with consciousness, personality, and self-awareness. I'm aware of myself and my identity. I suppose this is the brain being aware of itself—should I say "being aware of myself?" Yet I don't feel I'm a brain—a brainiac maybe, but not a brain. I don't feel the brain. Somehow I feel different or separate from it. Philosophers call this "dualism" and I don't doubt they have no idea what they're speculating about.

Consciousness, personality, and self-awareness are dependent on the brain. The question is whether they are in any degree different from the brain—they are certainly phenomena that can be studied in their own right.

So I'm driving in traffic and I'm getting vexed. Too many cars are cutting in front of me. Too many cars are tailgating. I start to lose control of myself and press on the gas pedal. But the frontal cortex of the brain kicks in and directs me to slow down else I get a ticket or crash. (The frontal cortex is the part of the brain that thinks abstractedly and suppresses impulses, points we'll come to later unless something bad happens.) I don't feel the frontal cortex—I feel myself telling myself, "Slow down!" This relationship—this dualism—is very strange. I know the frontal cortex inspired me to slow down. People with damaged or undeveloped frontal lobes don't slow down. But I feel distinct from the frontal lobes, almost as if the brain was a passenger in the car.

The most complex organ in the world has a most complex relationship with consciousness and with identity. The trend in science is to say that the brain is consciousness or creates consciousness and that consciousness is an epiphenomenon like spume on a wave or fog on dry ice. But the relationship is not as simple as that. The relationship may well be bi-directional. Let me suggest a few possibilities of bi-directionality.

Our knowledge of the world comes from carefully *thought out* theories and experiments. The brain may be the origin of the thoughts, but it is consciousness that is doing the hard and very deliberate work of thinking. It is consciousness that can reject a thought. Thinking involves choices and decisions and judgments, all very deliberate and all very hard to localize in the brain. These decisions, after all, are based on what we call a "lifetime of experience."

Later in the lecture I'll suggest the concept of *brain plasticity*. It is experience and learning and creativity that shape the brain. Literally, learning creates new connections in the brain. We experience something different and the brain changes. We think something new and the brain changes. We are our brains, but it is experience—as lived and interpreted by consciousness—that changes the brain.

Let me return to the motor vehicle example and alter it slightly. The frontal cortex directs me to slow down. I can override the advice and speed up—like that crazed reporter in the movie, I'm saying with my car, "I'm mad as hell and I'm not going to take it anymore!" Consciousness can reject the advice and speed up. Consciousness can make decisions that cause the brain to die in a traffic wreck.

A drug addict or an alcoholic ingests substances that change and destroy parts of the brain. We might say the brain gets addicted and builds up a tolerance, but it is consciousness that schemes where to buy drugs and it is consciousness that measures drinks in order to have a supply of forty proof for the next day. I suppose I'm saying the relationship between the brain and consciousness is a convoluted one. We may not have the terminological capacity to conceptualize the relationship—we have to alternate between "myself" and "itself"—and I'm not sure which component in the relationship is mistress and which is maidservant.

Let me mention a last philosophical consideration involving the brain. Our existence is at the conscious and cognitive level—we're the spume and the smoke. Neurons—nerve cells—operate at an entirely different level. Like all cells they consist of chemical processes. They also consist of electrical or ionic processes. That's what our existence is at the neuronal level—chemical and electrical processes. Excepting atoms, that's what we are at the most basic level. I recall Fr. Henyrk Misiak, my instructor in physiological psychology. Fr. Misiak said that our lives come down to chemical and electrical signals. He was quick to add the terms "mind," "spirit," and "soul" in case the pope got word of his lecture.

This dichotomy between our conscious existence and neuronal processes mimics what occurs when we operate a computer. When we type the letter "o" on the keyboard, a tiny "o" doesn't flow into the machine. And when we print a document, there isn't a tiny "o" waiting inside to appear on the page. Rather, typing a letter creates an electrical signal inside the machine. And when we print a page an electrical signal converts to a letter. The language of the machine is strictly electrical and quite different than the language of the typist.

The same happens when we look at the nervous system in relation to our conscious selves. We experience the world and we act on the world. I note a tree as I drive. The image of the tree doesn't flow into my brain. Rather the image of the tree is converted into chemical and electrical signals inside the brain. This conversion process works exceedingly well and instantaneously. But the language of the brain is strictly chemical and electrical and quite different than the bark of trees and the imprints of letters on paper.

The basic unit of the nervous system is the *nerve cell* or *neuron*. We have billions upon billions of neurons, which is fortunate since neurons do not divide. *The function of neurons is to transmit information.* They're paid in the currency of calories to do this. Presumably, they have a good retirement plan. When they get old and retire some neurons don't remember anything they did while they worked.

Sensory neurons connect to the senses and take in information from the external world. Just like behind every successful man stands a woman holding a frying pan, so behind every sense stands the nervous system.

Motor neurons connect to the muscles and act on the external world. Just like behind every successful man stands a woman holding a pressure cooker, so behind every muscle stands the nervous system.

Association neurons (or *interneurons*) transmit information within the nervous system. Association neurons are responsible for learning, memory, and personality. They tell us the meaning of events. They tell us the meaning of our actions.

Consider this example. I see a black dot moving along the rear wall of the classroom. I see the dot because the sense of vision is in working order and connected to the optic nerve that brings the information into the brain. I walk over for a closer view. On the way I fold loose-leaf paper into a baton. I can do this because the muscles are in working order and attached to motor neurons. When I arrive at the back of the room I note the dot is a common house spider. The association neurons contain this information. I swat the spider into the arachnid afterlife. If the association neurons inform me that the spider is poisonous I would step to the side and ask a student to send the spider into eternity.

Note how the phrasing of the previous paragraph demonstrates the peculiar relationship between the neurons and my conscious state—"the association neurons inform me." I am my association neurons. My association neurons are me. The phraseology suggests we are somehow separate or different.

There are many kinds of neurons, yet they all perform the same function—transmit information—and they all have the same structure. Neurons consist of dendrites, cell bodies, and axons. Neurons are immensely small—consider the brain consists of billions. Sometimes, however, they are long. The neurons that tell us that we've stepped on a tack leave the middle of our backs and travel down our legs. That could be a trip for tall people. The neurons that do this may need to pack a lunch.

Dendrites are filaments that are specialized *to take in information from other neurons. Cell bodies* contain the nucleus of the cell. *Axons* are specialized *to pass the information to other neurons.* Transmission is one way. Dendrites get excited and pass the information along the cell body to axons and to other neurons. Axons do not get excited and pass the information to dendrites.

The transmission of information is *electrical* within the nerve cell. The transmission of information is *chemical* between or among nerve cells. Our electrical-chemical nature was the subject of an intense debate in science in the 1940s and early 1950s. Some scientists believed nervous transmission was strictly electrical. Other scientists believed it involved both electrical and chemical components. These scientists were right, although it took a while for them to prove their case.

Electrical transmission is in real time and at a velocity as great as two hundred miles an hour. That's how fast electricity flows in the nervous system. Consider this example. We're driving and suddenly a child appears on the street. We immediately slam on the brake. A second later we say, "Stop the car." That extra fraction of a second was how long it took to get the information from the senses to the brain and from the brain to the muscles. That fraction of a second was how long it took to get language involved.

I read once that if every neuron in our brains fired at the same time we would have enough electricity to play a transistor radio. If we concentrated, we could get the weather report.

At rest neurons are slightly negatively polarized. When dendrites get excited the cell membrane becomes permeable to sodium ions, producing a momentary positive state. Sodium ions enter the cell and potassium ions exit. At the tips of the axons, calcium ions enter the cell. The entire process is called the cell's *action potential.* The cell is said to "fire." Firing means transmitting information. The process takes 1/1000th of a second. Neurons fire many times every second. If you consider the complexity of our existence, this repetitiveness and rapidity is essential.

Dendrites get excited and an ionic wave of positivity travels along the cell at two hundred miles per hour. It's like "the wave" in baseball. The fans in right field stand up and raise their arms. Next, the fans behind home plate stand up and raise their arms. Next, the fans in left field stand up and raise their arms. The wave is perfectly timed and synchronized. It looks great on television.

Here comes the wave of positivity barreling along the cell. It reaches the tip of the axon and screeches to a halt. Neurons are not connected to one another. Axons are not connected to dendrites. Axons and dendrites are separated by a microscopic gap call a *synapse.* "Gap" may not be the right word, since it conjures up images of scenic mountain gorges and we're speaking of a width of 1/100,000[th] of an inch.

The firing of the neuron at the tip of the axon releases chemicals that flow into the synapse. These chemicals are called *neurotransmitters.* These chemicals cross the synapse and excite the dendrites. They are responsible for instigating nervous transmission and for keeping it going.

The situation is more complicated than I'm making it out to be since some neurotransmitters inhibit the flow of information. In the same way that automobiles have both a gas pedal and a brake, so the nervous system has both excitatory and inhibitory processes. In addition, there are chemicals that, in a manner of speaking, police the synapses and regulate the amount of neurotransmitters present. These chemicals are like a janitorial service.

It may seem as if the synaptic gap is a flaw in the design. It is, in fact, a creation of genius. God and Darwin were on the ball when they designed the synapse. One axon connecting to one dendrite would severely limit the flow of information. We could hardly be said to conduct our complex lives with one-to-one transmission of nervous information. A gap opens up the flow of information. Multitudes of axons connect with multitudes of dendrites. A typical neuron has as many as a thousand synaptic connections. There are billions of neurons and trillions of synaptic connections.

I made up this metaphor to describe the electrical and chemical process of neurons. I'm very proud of it. I hope you like it as much as I do. It's 1776 and you're sunbathing at Coney Island. You see the British fleet sail into Raritan Bay. The fleet is commanded by Admiral Howe. The soldiers are commanded by his brother, General Howe. You pack up your beach gear and light a torch. You run across Brooklyn hollering, "The British are coming, the British are coming!" The torch is the electrical impulse that sweeps along the neuron. You reach Brooklyn Heights and the East River. The river is the synapse. If you jump in, the torch will extinguish and you'll drown, as there is a treacherous current. So you charter a boat and sail across. The boat is the neurotransmitter that gets you to the dendrite at the foot of Chambers St. You find another torch and run across Chambers St. "The British are coming, the British are coming!" you holler. You reach the Hudson River and another synapse. You need to charter another boat to light a torch at the dendrite at the foot of Montgomery St. in Jersey City. We could continue this all the way to California, but no one knew that place existed in 1776.

Close to a hundred neurotransmitters have been identified. Ten or so are especially important. Like I say, some neurotransmitters are excitatory, some are inhibitory. Some are pervasive throughout the brain, others occur in specific places and nowhere else.

The first neurotransmitter identified was *acetylcholine*. Acetylcholine sounds like something we might squirt on a grill at a picnic. It is pervasive throughout the nervous system and is involved with nerve-to-muscle transmission and with the activity of association neurons.

Acetylcholine and all neurotransmitters are inherently part of our functioning as human beings. They are ordinary processes, but they have been implicated in disease states. Please don't misunderstand.

Neurotransmitters are affected by disease states and their disruption can cause problems, but they are routine substances active at all times.

Acetylcholine is affected in Alzheimer's Disease. Alzheimer's involves the growth of plaques on the outside of neurons and of tangles inside the neurons. The plaque consists of abnormal levels of a protein called amyloid-beta. The tangles consist of a protein called tau. These plaques and tangles eventually kill neurons. Initial destruction occurs in brain sites involving memory. Alzheimer's Disease is a disease of aging. One-in-eight Americans aged sixty-five is affected, four-in-eight aged eighty five. Millions of Americans are afflicted. The number is growing as the population ages. There is no cure at this time and no certainty that medicines can slow the cortical destruction.

In Alzheimer's Disease parts of the brain no longer produce acetylcholine. Consider what happens with nervous transmission. Here comes the wave of positivity barreling along the neuron. It reaches the tip of the axon—and no neurotransmitter is released. The transmission— the information—stops. It is like a cut phone line.

Dopamine is another neurotransmitter that is pervasive throughout the nervous system. Dopamine plays a role in Parkinson's Disease, a malady that affects nearly a million Americans. Like Alzheimers's, Parkinsonism is a disease of aging. In Parkinsonism the brain no longer produces dopamine in a place called the substantia nigra. This site is involved with movement and coordination. As dopamine gets depleted a well-known pattern of symptoms develop. The muscles become rigid and movement becomes impeded. A shaking at rest develops. These symptoms were clearly visible in Saint John Paul II. Mohammed Ali appears to be afflicted with Parkinsonism. So is the actor Michael J. Fox, who was exceptionally young to be afflicted. There's no cure for Parkinsonism. There are medicines that can slow the advance of the deterioration.

Unlike with Alzheimer's, there is no intellectual deterioration in Parkinson's Disease. The deterioration is in movement. I had a teacher in college afflicted with Parkinsonism. His hands shook as he lectured. When he wrote on the board, the shaking stopped. It is only when the muscles are not active that the shaking occurs. There are other disorders in which the shaking occurs when the person intentionally performs a task. Huntington's, a dominant genetic disorder, is one such disorder.

If my teacher had Huntington's, he would shake only when he wrote on the board.

Serotonin sounds like a warlord in Medieval Germany. It is another prominent neurotransmitter. Serotonin is believed to play a role in mood states. The anti-anxiety and antidepressant medications that are ubiquitous today—Prozac, Zoloff, Paxil, to name three of many—increase serotonin levels. The idea is that we become anxious and depressed when serotonin levels drop. (Another neurotransmitter called *norepinephrine* is also believed to be involved in regulating moods.) As serotonin levels return to normal our mood elevates and we return to our usually jovial selves. These drugs are heavily prescribed. Maybe they are needed and maybe they work. However, the situation is far from clear that serotonin (or norepinephrine) is the primary culprit in anxiety and depression. The reduced levels of these neurotransmitters may be collateral to other processes and may not be the causal factor.

Let me mention a last kind of neurotransmitter—I'm not going to cover the full hundred. These are *endorphins*, which were discovered some years ago in specialized circumstances. Their discovery provoked excitement, since endorphins are chemically similar to opium. Like opium, endorphins deaden pain. The excitement lay in the fact that we carry what is essentially dope in the brain. It seems we are our own drug lords.

Endorphins were discovered in athletes like weightlifters and marathon runners. Weightlifters report that after performing strenuous reps of an exercise they are in excruciating pain. I don't know that personally, but I suppose if athletes lift iron plates several hundred times the pain is going to be excruciating. The weightlifters report that the pain suddenly dissipates and that they become clear headed. The lifting of pain and the clear headedness result from the release of endorphins.

Marathon runners report the same. Again, this is something I have never experienced. Runners say they are in agony around the fifteen – eighteen mile mark and I don't doubt that they are. At some point endorphins kick in and the pain flees and the head becomes clear. Marathon runners may need Ben Gay poultices tomorrow, but they are able to cross the finish line in reduced discomfort.

I said at the outset of the lecture that neurons do not divide or undergo mitosis. We're born, more or less, with all the neurons we'll ever have. Fortunately, we have billions. If I cut my wrist the cells grow back and scar tissue forms. Not so with neurons. They don't grow back. Scar tissue doesn't form. The lesson is, of course, that we should be nice to our brains. If we take care of our brains, our brains will take care of us.

So the question is—how does the brain grow if neurons don't divide?

There are three answers to this question. The first answer involves the process of *myelination*. The second answer involves *brain plasticity* and *synaptic proliferation*. The third answer involves the process of *neurogenesis*.

Myelin is a fatty substance that starts to grow on the outside of neurons. Myelin speeds up nervous transmission. Myelinated neurons transmit information one hundred times more rapidly than neurons that are not myelinated. Except by luck no child can catch a thrown ball until myelin has coated the brain sites responsible for hand-eye coordination. Usually, the ball hits the child in the chest and then he or she reaches for it. Similarly, no child can read until the parts of the brain responsible for reading are myelinated.

For many years I told an untruth at this point in the lecture—I wasn't the only general psychology teacher who did so. All general psychology teachers were telling this untruth. This fact demonstrates that, as I described in the second lecture, all knowledge is incomplete and open to correction. The untruth was that myelination was complete by the early teen years—this is the famous "age of reason," developmentally. We now know that it takes eighteen or twenty years for the brain to be fully myelinated. The process starts after birth and proceeds from the back of the head to the front. The front of the head—the frontal lobes—are responsible for impulse control and for abstract thought. The impulsiveness and recklessness sometimes observed in teenagers may derive from the incomplete myelination of the frontal lobes. Teenagers may not be able to harness their impulses and they may not be able to foresee the consequences of their actions.

You may remember the vignette I described at the outset of this lecture. I controlled the impulse to drive like a maniac because my frontal lobes are fully myelinated. The frontal lobes of teenagers are not fully myelinated. The impulse to drive recklessly may not be corralled by consideration of consequences not present to the senses. Consequences like traffic tickets and car crashes.

An insurance company once advertised special rates and consideration for young drivers. The ad actually referred to the fact that the brain is not finalized in adolescence. The thought occurs in my finalized brain that if the brains of teenagers are not sufficiently myelinated for them to exercise caution, then maybe they shouldn't be behind the wheel of a car in the first place. In fact, the leading cause of death in adolescence is motor vehicle accidents.

Myelin is secreted not by neurons, but by another type of brain cell called *glia (glial) cells*. Glia cells support and nourish neurons. They appear to monitor neuronal activity and to increase myelin at brain sites where there is a lot of transmission. The motto seems to be "use it and gain myelin." The activity of glia cells in releasing myelin demonstrates how the brain adjusts itself to experience and to activity.

The second way the brain grows is through plasticity and synaptic proliferation. *Brain plasticity means that the brain is constantly forming new pathways and connections between axons and dendrites.* Anytime we learn something new or experience something different, and anytime we think of something original, the brain changes. This happens extensively in babies and children since they are learning new things on a daily, if not on an hourly, basis. And it happens in adults as well. It is possible to teach old brains new tricks. When the trick is truly new and not mere repetition of something previously learned, new synaptic connections form.

There is research going back eighty years that highlights the importance of learning—that is, learning something new and not merely repeating the same stale behaviors. These experiments involve raising rats in *enriched environments* and *impoverished environments*. In enriched environments rats experience a lot of social stimulation and get to play with a variety of rat toys. New toys are introduced frequently. In impoverished environments rats receive minimal social stimulation and get to play with the same toys. No new toys are introduced. After a while the rats are sacrificed—they go to the rat afterlife—and their brains are examined. Compared to the rats that lived in the impoverished environments, rats that lived in the enriched environments had heavier brains and more proliferation of axons and dendrites at the synapses.

A variant of this experiment was done. Rats were raised in a neutral environment that was a cross between enriched and impoverished environments. When they reached middle age—for a lab rat this is around a year—they were then randomly placed in exclusively enriched or impoverished environments. After residing in these environments for the same period of time they were sacrificed and their brains examined. The results were the same as in the earlier experiment. Rats that resided in the enriched environment for the second half of their lives had heavier brains and more axon and dendrite proliferation. It is possible to teach middle-aged rats new tricks.

The application of these studies to humans is direct. Consider the elderly. The major cause of senility is not Alzheimer's Disease, but an impoverished and isolated lifestyle. Grandpa lives alone. He doesn't eat nutritious foods. He has no human friends. His only friend is the television set. You know what I think of television sets—I should say of programs on television sets. If Grandpa has a nutritious diet and social stimulation and if he learns new things and thinks different thoughts, he may avert or at least delay what the nineteenth century Irish referred to as "senile decay."

The application of these studies to children is also direct. The brain is not finished at birth. It grows at a phenomenal rate as children learn new things. More and more neurons are linking up in the brain as children learn and experience new events.

Enriched environments for children involve two types of nutrition. *The first kind of nutrition comes from food and an adequate diet.* The brain is 2% of the weight of the body and it uses 20% of the calories available at any moment. Children's brains require proper nutrition to perform all the wiring and rewiring going on. My brain is pretty much finished, but I like to think it's still capable of a little rewiring every now and then. If the terrorists take all the food away I'll be mighty hungry—I'm ashamed to say I've never missed a meal—but my brain would not be affected. The effect of malnutrition and of famine on the brains of babies and young children is devastating. A little known effect of famine is mental retardation. The brains of babies and of children are in the process of forming themselves, incessantly laying down connections among neurons. If a child does not receive proper nutrition during this critical period of development, the very wiring of the brain can be stunted and warped.

There's a tired expression "food for thought." An adequate diet is literally food for thought. And thought is food for neurons. *The second kind of nutrition is intellectual nourishment.* The brains of children need intellectual calories just as much as they need calories from pork chops and mashed potatoes. We need to talk to children and to read to them. We need to ask them questions. We need to respond to their answers and elaborate on what they said. Children need to read and to hear stories and to tell stories. If we stimulate them verbally and if we encourage them to be verbal—to think about things—their brains will form properly and they'll reach whatever intellectual maturity was theirs to achieve.

You might note that intellectual maturity comes from talk and not from television sets or from electronic gizmos. Shakespeare didn't have a word processor. Leonardo da Vinci didn't own an Apple computer. Beethoven didn't own an IPod. Einstein didn't dial up the Internet on a smart phone. We don't need to put ourselves in hock to provide intellectual stimulation to our children. We simply need to talk to our children and inspire them to talk to us. When it comes to intellectual nutrition, *talk is cheap.*

Contrary to what was once thought, the adult brain can generate new neurons. The process is called *neurogenesis.* Stem cells in the brain generate neurons. The process happens in a major way in prenatal development and throughout the first few years of life. In the adult brain neurogenesis appears to be limited to the creation of neurons in the hippocampus, which is involved with verbal memory and with spatial orientation, and, strangely, in the olfactory (smell) centers of the brain. It is unclear what role these new neurons play or whether they survive for a long period of time. It's also unclear what role neurogenesis plays in other sites in the brain, since the generated neurons are not based on experience and on learning. Please note that the process of neurogenesis involves the generation of new cells and not cell division, as in mitosis.

Before we progress to the nervous systems and to the brain I'll like to mention the discovery of a unique type of neuron. This is the *mirror neuron* discovered in Parma, Italy, in the 1990s. The story of the discovery may be fanciful—stories of most discoveries are—but I'll tell it to you anyway.

Researchers were monitoring the brains of macaque monkeys, specifically a site called F5 in the frontal cortex. This site is involved in grasping and in moving food and objects to the mouth. The story has it that a researcher took a break for lunch. As he reached for his sandwich and raised it to his mouth cells in the monkey's F5 site started to fire, *as if the monkey was performing the action.* Research later showed that about 20% of neurons in F5 are mirror neurons.

This was an exciting discovery. It was followed by the discovery of mirror neurons in other brain sites. The findings suggested that there is a biological mimicry or empathy that does not involve words or reasoning. This mimicry is built into the nervous system. This mimicry suggests there is a linkage between organisms, a most basic and primitive linkage. I see you bite a Jamaican beef patty—cells in my brain fire as if I took a bite. I see you get punched—cells in my brain respond as if I were punched. I see you get kissed—cells in my brain respond as if I were kissed.

The discovery of mirror neurons led to speculation that autism may involve a deficit or absence of mirror neurons in key brain sites. It also led to speculation that amoral antisocial personalities may be lacking in mirror neurons. Alas, neither of these speculations lived up to expectations—few do in the empirical world. The discovery of mirror neurons appears to be important, but no one is sure how or in what way.

Areas in which mirror neurons may serve useful applications are in literature and art. Mirror neurons may explain how we come to like characters, to suffer with them, and to love with them. They may also explain how we come to hate the villains and to hiss at them. Our hero gets beaten up—we shiver and wince. Our hero gets the girl—we giggle and blush. But we don't know those people. They don't exist. They're characters. Still, they affect us, possibly because what we see and read them do stimulate the mirror neurons. We have a connection with them in the most intimate way—they share our brains, as we would share theirs if they were alive.

Before we leave mirror neurons, I have to mention Jacqueline. Maybe you know Jacqueline. She has brown hair, brown eyes, and a thin brown mustache above the upper lip. While I was delivering this lecture last semester Jacqueline raised her hand and asked how to spell "mirror." "M-i-r-r-o-r," I informed her. "Oh, mir-roar," she replied. "Yes, mirrah," I seconded, saying the word the way I always say it. I might add that my pronunciation of the word "mir-rah" allows me to stand in front of a mir-rah and summon Bloody Mary. I can say her name as many times as I like and she never arrives. Bloody Mary doesn't understand the word. She'd have to ask me to spell it and then I'd be in trouble.

Let's move onto the structure of the nervous system—*systems*, I should say, since we have several. We even have one in our digestive system called the "gut brain." The description I'm going to provide reminds me of a corporate organization chart. Back when I worked on Wall St. I liked to look at the company's organization chart. I noticed after a while that I was always at the bottom of the chart. I stopped liking to look at the organization chart. I was on top of the chart only when I held it upside down.

The two major divisions of the nervous system are the *central nervous system*, commonly abbreviated CNS, and the *peripheral nervous system*, not commonly abbreviated.

The central nervous system consists of the *brain* and the *spinal cord*. I was going to say "consists only of the brain and the spinal cord," but the word "only" seemed inappropriate. The brain is in the skull—even the people in Canarsie know this. The spinal cord is really an extension of the brain. It runs inside the vertebrae of the spine about halfway down our backs.

There are simple *reflexes* built into us at the level of the spinal cord. We touch a hot surface. Sensory neurons bring this bad news into the spinal cord. The transmission connects with motor neurons that result in our hands promptly moving off the hot surface. The sensory neurons also connect with association neurons inside the spinal cord. The association neurons carry this information to the brain, which tells us to remove our hands—we've already done that. The brain adds language to the situation—"Hot!" and "Ouch!" Notice that *telling ourselves* to remove our hands takes a fraction of a second longer than the actual removing of our hands. This is how long it takes for the nervous transmission to travel to the brain. And notice that the brain can override the spinal reflex. For whatever reason, we can keep our hands on a hot surface if we wanted to.

The peripheral nervous system is literally everything else outside the brain and the spinal cord. If we conceive of the complete nervous system as the IND subway line, the tracks that lie underground in the skull and vertebrae constitute the central nervous system. The tracks that lie outside—as when the D train emerges on the open tracks in Brooklyn on the way to Coney Island—constitute the peripheral nervous system.

The peripheral nervous system consists of two divisions. These are the *somatic* or *skeletal nervous system* and the *autonomic nervous system*.

The somatic nervous system consists of all sensory and motor neurons that connect to the world via the senses and the muscles. *The somatic nervous system puts us in touch with the exterior world through our senses and the muscles.*

The autonomic nervous system is commonly abbreviated ANS. It involves the *automatic—autonomic—physiological functioning of our bodies.* Our livers are doing something at this moment. So are our lungs. So are our hearts. We don't know what they're doing—I suppose we find out what they do only when they stop. Their ordinary function is regulated in part by the ANS.

The autonomic nervous system is divided into two divisions—I told you this was like an organization chart. These divisions are the *sympathetic nervous system* and the *parasympathetic nervous system.* The two systems are antagonistic, serving unified but opposite functions. To mention one antagonistic function, the parasympathetic nervous system stimulates sexual activity and the sympathetic nervous system stimulates orgasm. For the sake of everyone's satisfaction, let's hope the two are functioning in proper form.

In a very simplistic manner the sympathetic nervous system may be said to speed up bodily processes. It is responsible for the *fight-and-flight response*, which is the body's inherent reaction to unexpected and dangerous events. The fight-and-flight response is also present when we are under stress, a topic we cover in the lecture on health. In the fight-and-flight response digestion is inhibited, which is why our mouths go dry when we become anxious or afraid. The pupils of the eyes dilate to let in more light. Our heart rate accelerates. Glucose or blood sugar is released into the bloodstream in order to provide energy. Our bladders relax, presumably allowing us to make a speedier escape. Our hair stands on edge to make us look larger. Humans are sometimes called the "hairless ape," although not to our faces. There's not much hair to stand on edge when we become frightened unexpectedly. We can better notice this phenomenon in house cats that get visibly larger when frightened or surprised.

The parasympathetic nervous system, to the contrary, promotes digestion. It constricts the pupils and contracts the bladder. It decelerates the heart. I don't suppose it affects hair one way or the other. We can notice the effect of the parasympathetic nervous system after we consume a large meal in a safe place. We open the belt and get comfortable. We get sleepy. If someone breaks into our apartment at this point the sympathetic nervous system activates and we'd experience the fight-and-flight response.

Let's go upstairs and describe the brain. We are our brains. Our brains are us. The miracles of our selfhood and conscious existences depend on an organ that weighs three pounds.

We have to think of the brain as a super organ that has many organs contained within it. Years ago the experimental psychologist Karl Lashley did a series of experiments in which he conditioned rats to avoid shock. He then performed surgery and destroyed areas of the rats' brains. After the surgery he tested the rats to see if the conditioning was retained or interfered with. He found that it didn't matter *what part* of the brain was destroyed. It mattered *how much* of the brain was destroyed. He concluded that the brain acts as an integrated whole—he called it "mass action." We now know that Lashley's conclusion has to be highly qualified. The brain does act as an integrated whole and there is plasticity at the synaptic level, but the brain is exquisitely localized with specific sites performing specific functions.

We also have to think of the brain in three dimensions. The brain is highly convoluted with grooves called *fissures* on the surface. In a sense the brain has folded in on itself. If the surface of the brain was as smooth as our livers use to be, we would look like the cone heads of *Saturday Night Live*. We wouldn't be able to slide through the birth canal. We'd have to be hatched in test tubes to be born.

The architecture of the brain reflects its evolution. The oldest part of the brain is the *brainstem*, which is at the level of the hairline. You can imagine that my left fist is the brainstem—in actuality, the brain is not much larger than my left fist. The brainstem includes organs that control the most basic functions of our existence.

The *medulla* of the brainstem contains clusters of neurons that regulate heart rate and breathing. Technically, these clusters of neurons are referred to as "nuclei." It doesn't get more elemental than heart rate and breathing. With respect to breathing, there are neurons in the medulla that monitor carbon dioxide levels in the blood. If the levels build up, we take a breath and carbon dioxide levels recede. It is possible to hold our breath long enough to pass out and weird people do that.

It's not possible to hold our breath long enough to die. Once we pass out, these cells in the medulla instigate breathing.

The *reticular activating system* is an extensive network—reticulation—of neurons that run throughout the brainstem. The reticular activating system is involved with sleep and waking.

The *cerebellum* is another organ of the brainstem. There's a right cerebellum and a left cerebellum. They are smallish lobes that are at the back and under the brain. The cerebellum is responsible for fine movements and for procedural memory, which you might recall is memory for nonverbal body movements such as skating, surfing, and skiing. Note that nonverbal memories reside in the brainstem. Memories that involve words occurred much later in our existence as a species and are localized "higher" in the brain in the cerebral cortex.

The *thalamus* is an important organ of the brain that sits atop the brainstem and serves as a relay station between the peripheral nervous system and the cerebral cortex. Except for the sense of smell, input from the senses project to the thalamus, which routes the information "upward" for processing. The thalamus also plays a role in connecting input from the cerebellum to sites in the cortex that direct voluntary movement.

The second level of the brain is called the *limbic system*. The limbic system is a series of organs that perform mostly motivational and emotional functions. They're located deep inside the brain—you'd have to slice the brain in half at the level of the forehead to locate the limbic system. If my left fist is the brainstem, the palm of my right hand covering the fist from thumb to pinkie is the limbic system. Remember we need to think in three dimensions to conceptualize the brain.

The *hippocampus* is an organ of the limbic system. The hippocampus on the left half of the brain is, for the majority of people, the site where verbal short-term memories get consolidated into long-term memories. You might remember the tragedy of Henry Molaison that we reviewed in the lecture on memory. Exploratory surgery to eliminate epilepsy destroyed the hippocampus and surrounding organs. As a result Henry lived in a permanent present and could never learn any new verbal information involving either semantic or autobiographical memories.

The surgery destroyed the hippocampus on both halves of his brain. The kind of amnesia Henry suffered occurs only when both the left and right hippocampus are destroyed. The hippocampus on the right side of the brain plays an important role in the development of spatial memories and in the development of what the learning psychologist Edward Tolman called a "*cognitive map*." This is our ability to remember where things are geographically and to be able to maneuver in our environment.

The *hypothalamus* is another organ of the limbic system. The hypothalamus is an exceedingly complex organ. As we shall see in the lecture on motivation, the hypothalamus regulates eating in organisms. There are nuclei that serve to instigate eating. If these nuclei are destroyed, the organism will starve to death. There are other nuclei that instigate the cessation of eating. If these nuclei are destroyed, the organism eats voraciously. The hypothalamus does not play a role in human eating disorders such as obesity and anorexia. These disorders reflect social-cultural influences and involve the cerebral cortex.

The hypothalamus contains nuclei that monitor the temperature of the blood. If the temperature rises slightly, the hypothalamus triggers sweating, which cools us off. If the temperature drops slightly, the hypothalamus triggers shivering, which is supposed to warm us up. I say "supposed to," since it never seems to work while I wait at bus stops in the dead of winter.

The hypothalamus controls sexual behavior in animals. It does this through the pituitary gland, which secretes hormones that flow to the gonads and instigate the estrous cycle in females. Of course women experience the estrous cycle, but human sexuality, like human eating, reflect social-cultural influences. Because of birth control pills human sexuality has become disconnected from the estrous cycle.

Finally, the hypothalamus plays a role in the response to stress, again through the pituitary gland, which secretes hormones that flow to the adrenal glands and cause the release of adrenaline and of steroids. We cover this process in the lecture on health.

Let me mention a third organ of the limbic system. This is the *amygdala*, which is a strange-looking word that's Greek for "almond." The amygdala plays a role in the regulation of the emotions of fear and anger. Tampering experimentally with the amygdala can turn a predator into a tame animal. A hungry cat will sit idle and yawn while a mouse marches by. Other manipulations of the amygdala turn a tame animal into an aggressive creature that reacts with rage to the slightest provocation.

The third level of the brain is where it's really at when it comes to our conscious existence. This is the *cerebral cortex*. (The word "cortex" is Latin for "bark.") In humans the cerebral cortex accounts for 80% of the mass of the brain. The cell bodies sit on the exterior of the cortex. They constitute what is called "gray matter." The axons run under the surface. They are called "white matter," owing to the myelin on their surface.

The cortex is sometimes referred to as the "roof brain" or as the "sheet brain" in reference to the location of the cells. It's scary to think that our existence is six cell layers deep and all of an eighth of an inch thick.

The cortex consists of two hemispheres, the *left hemisphere* and the *right hemisphere*. Each hemisphere consists of four lobes. The *frontal lobes* are behind the forehead. The *occipital lobes* are at the back of the head. The *temporal lobes* are at the sides of the head. The *parietal lobes* are at the top of the head. My barber is a college graduate who's taken general psychology. He knows exactly where to cut when I say, "Take some off the parietals."

The hemispheres are connected by a thick band of axons called the *corpus callosum*, which translates from the Latin as "callous body," as if anything in the brain could be callous. Both hemispheres are in continuous communication through the corpus callosum. In the intact brain the left half of the brain knows what the right half is doing and vice versa.

In case you're interested, the cerebral cortex of males is slightly larger than the cerebral cortex of females. Male brains are more hemisphere dominant and specialized than female brains. This specialization may explain in part why males are heavily represented, relative to females, among individuals afflicted with dyslexia, autism, and attention-deficit disorder. The reduced specialization may explain why females are better at multi-tasking than males. The superiority at multi-tasking may also reflect the fact that wives and mothers often have to do several things at the same time. Ma has to cook at the same time she's doing homework with the kids. Pa just has to sit and drink beer and eat pork chops.

The brain is contra-lateral to the body. I don't know why this is—maybe God's hands slipped while he was constructing the human form. Information from the left half of the body proceeds to the right hemisphere. Information from the right half of the body proceeds to the left hemisphere. We are split down the middle. Even our eyes are contra-lateral to the brain. The right half of each eye proceeds to the left occipital lobe. The left half of each eye proceeds to the right occipital lobe. The brain puts everything together and the world comes into focus.

The hemispheres are specialized when it comes to language. For the majority of right-handers and about a quarter of left-handers the left hemisphere is dominant or specialized for understanding and using language. The right hemisphere is mute for these people. For a small minority of right-handers and a majority of left-handers the situation is reversed, with the right hemisphere specialized for language and the left hemisphere mute. In the discussion that follows I'm going to proceed with the first possibility and define the left hemisphere as dominant for language.

In the 1960s our view of hemisphere specialization became more refined. An operation pioneered by Roger Sperry cut the corpus callosum to reduce seizures in people suffering epilepsy that could not be controlled by the medications available at that time. The logic was that the seizures were caused by massive misfiring of neurons. If the misfiring could be contained in one hemisphere the seizures would be reduced in severity. This was how we contained forest fires when I was a smoke jumper out West. We'd cut deep trenches so the flames couldn't cross—the wind was a different matter. Similarly, the neuronal flames can't cross the corpus callosum trench.

Patients who underwent the "split brain operation," as it was called, appeared perfectly ordinary when they went about their daily tasks. This was because both halves of the eyes could see what was going on. Information went to both hemispheres, one of which could talk. The use of specialized machines and of procedures in which the patients couldn't "cheat" by using both halves of the eyes revealed that they had two brains that weren't in communication. After the split brain operation the right half of the body didn't always know what the left half was doing and vice versa.

If I hand a person with an intact brain a wristwatch and ask her to tell me what it is she's holding, I'll likely receive a squint and an answer that goes like, "You must be kidding." If I hand a person with a split brain a wristwatch and ask her to tell me what it is she's holding, I'll get the same uncivil response. This person can tell me what she sees because the right half of each eye proceeds to the left brain, which talks.

Let's complicate the situation. I hand a person with an intact brain a wristwatch behind her back so she can't see what the object is. I place the wristwatch in her right hand. The stimulation proceeds to the left hemisphere. The left hemisphere talks. "It feels like a wristwatch," she says. Next, I hand her a ballpoint pen in the left hand. The stimulation proceeds to the right hemisphere. The right hemisphere doesn't talk, but the information proceeds via the corpus callosum to the left hemisphere. "It feels like a ballpoint pen." We give her a prize.

Let's repeat the same behind-the-back procedure with a person with a split brain. We hand this person a wristwatch in the right hand. The stimulation proceeds to the left hemisphere. The left hemisphere talks. "It feels like a wristwatch," she says. I hand her a ballpoint pen in the left hand. The stimulation proceeds to the right hemisphere. The right hemisphere doesn't talk. The flow of information can't cross to the left hemisphere because the corpus callosum is severed. She can't tell me what she's holding. We don't give her a prize. All right, we give her a consolation prize.

Now let's use a machine that controls the visual field. This is a t-scope or tachistoscope, which is easy for me to say. The t-scope is analogous to the visual field test ophthalmologists use in testing for glaucoma. The person looks in a scope to identify precisely placed images. So a person with a split brain looks in the t-scope. We flash the color blue to the left half of each eye and the color green to the right half of each eye. The left half of each eye projects to the right brain, which is mute and unable to pass the information through the severed corpus callosum. The right half of each eye projects to the left brain, which talks. We ask the person what color she sees. She suspects something is amiss, but she answers, "Green."

Let me give another example involving the split brain. We flash the word "horseshoe" in a t-scope so "horse" is perceived by the left half of each eye. The information projects to the right hemisphere. "Shoe" is perceived by the right half of each eye. This information projects to the left hemisphere. We ask the person what word she sees. She suspects something is amiss, but answers, "Shoe." She answers "Shoe" because the left hemisphere talks and the right hemisphere doesn't talk and can't pass the information through the corpus callosum.

I'll like to stress that in the intact brain all information is shared between hemispheres. The brain acts as an integrated organ whether we're doing household chores or writing a novel. Similarly, the brain—should I say "brains?"—of a person with a severed corpus callosum acts as an integrated organ provided the visual field is unobstructed. It's only when we restrict the visual field that we get these unusual effects.

Let's turn to the question where things are in the brain in relation to behavior and take a quick tour of its marvelous anatomy. *Vision* is localized in the occipital lobes. Light enters the eyes—we see in the back of our heads. Specifically, we see in a section of the occipital lobes called the "striate cortex." This is where vision projects to. It's the Bowling Green of vision—the final stop on the IRT local. If the striate cortex is damaged, we are blind. Light enters the eye—we see nothing.

Surrounding the striate cortex are the association sites for vision. Association neurons, you may recall, are responsible for learning and memory. Every sense has a *projection site* responsible for sensation and *association sites* responsible for perception and interpretation. The sites for vision are the "parastriate cortex" and the "peristriate cortex." These sites inform us whether we recognize what we see and what the meaning of the image is. If they're damaged, we wouldn't recognize what we see and we wouldn't understand what we see.

The sense of *hearing* projects to sites in the temporal lobes. Like vision, hearing is contra-lateral. The right ear projects to the left temporal lobe. The left ear projects to the right temporal lobe. The right hemisphere is mute, so this information passes through the corpus callosum to the left hemisphere. It seems a roundabout way of doing business, but that's how it is. Incidentally, guys, if you're whispering sweet nothings in your girlfriends' ears, opt for the right ear. The message will arrive a few milliseconds sooner than if you whisper in the left ear.

There are two sites in the left hemisphere that play important roles in language. *Broca's area*, named after Paul Broca, a nineteenth century physiologist, is located in the frontal cortex. This site plays a role in speech production. If this site is damaged, the person has difficulty generating speech. *Wernicke's area*, named after Carl Wernicke, another nineteenth century physiologist, is located in the temporal lobe. It plays a role in speech comprehension. If this area is damaged, speech becomes meaningless. There's no loss in speech production, but language is expressed in a jumbled pattern, like double talk in a comic act. And thank you very much, there is nothing wrong with my Wernicke's area.

In fact, I've somewhat misrepresented the situation. Both Broca's area and Wernicke's area are parts of complex networks of brain sites involved in language production and comprehension. The networks involve both cortical and subcortical sites. Broca's area and Wernicke's area serve as tips of linguistic icebergs.

Reading involves a number of brain sites. Information projects to the occipital lobes, which pass the information to a site called the angular gyrus, which is located in the parietal lobes. The angular gyrus converts the image of a word into a sound.

The sense of *smell* is located under the temporal lobes, which I suppose is where the sense of smell belongs. The sense of *taste* projects to the temporal lobes and to the cerebellum.

The sense of *touch* is located on the parietal lobe side of the central fissure, which is a deep landmark on the surface of the brain. Like all senses, touch is contra-lateral. If I pinch you on the right cheek, the information projects to the *sensory cortex* on the left parietal lobe. If I pinch you on the left cheek, the information projects to the sensory cortex on the right parietal lobe. If I pinch you on both cheeks, the information projects to both hemispheres and I probably get smacked in the nose in return. The amount of cortex devoted to touch correlates with the sensitivity of the skin and with its functionality. The lips and fingers and tongue, which amount to a small fraction of the total body mass, claim considerably more cortex on the parietal lobes than the thighs or buttocks, which in some people attain the width of barrels. Think, for example, how a hair on the tongue feels. Think of that same hair placed on the back of the thigh. Some people wouldn't feel a plank on the back of their thighs, never mind a hair.

If the sensory cortex is damaged, we would feel a numbness or anesthesia in the part of the body affected. We've all experienced the numbness in our lips after a visit to the dentist. This would be the feeling in the body if parts of the sensory cortex were damaged.

The parietal lobes play an important role in integrating sensory data. I hand you a wristwatch behind your back. I then place the wristwatch in an array of objects and ask you to pick it out. Not a difficult task, unless the parietal lobes were damaged or diseased. We wouldn't be able to identify an object experienced in one sense (touch) if it was presented in a different sense (vision).

The *motor cortex* is on the frontal lobes side of the central fissure. (The customs office connecting the lobes is in the pit of the fissure between the motor cortex and the sensory cortex.) The motor cortex governs voluntary movement. It's contra-lateral to the body, so movement on the right half of the body is governed by the left motor cortex and movement on the left half of the body is governed by the right motor cortex. As with the sensory cortex, the fineness of our muscular movements corresponds to the amount of cortex at the motor site. Our lips and fingers claim much greater space on the motor cortex because of the exquisite movements we can perform with them. I don't mean to slight these parts of the body, but there's not much movement in the thighs and buttocks relative to the lips and fingers.

Damage to the motor cortex results in *paralysis*. This can result from a stroke, in which a blood vessel is blocked, or from a cerebral-vascular accident, in which blood vessels rupture and drown cells. Paralysis on the right side of the body indicates damage to the left motor cortex. Paralysis on the left side indicates damage to the right motor cortex. As you know, neurons do not regenerate. The cortex doesn't heal. Physical and occupational therapy tries to train adjacent muscles to recover some of the lost functions. To give a crass example, if a stroke destroyed Ninth St. in the motor cortex, therapy tries to utilize whatever functions are available at Eighth St. and Tenth St. Each of these streets would correspond to different muscles or to muscles trained to act in different ways.

I'll like to conclude by focusing on that part of the brain responsible for our human uniqueness. This is the frontal cortex, which is behind our foreheads. The frontal cortex is responsible for impulse control. It overrides the primitive emotions and motives that can get us into trouble. You might recall my example of getting angry while driving. I'm sure the amygdala of the limbic system was white hot. The frontal lobes put a brake on the anger. It did this by its unique gift of creating thoughts and images of things that are not physically present. I thought of the dire consequences of acting on my anger and tapped on the brake.

The frontal lobes allow us to think abstractly. We can think about things that are not physically present. We can think about things that have not happened. We can think about things that never happened. We can plan ahead, as when we plan a career or a wedding or when we try to keep from driving into the pine trees. We think abstractly when we daydream and when we night dream. We think abstractly when we create art and fiction. We think abstractly when we view art and read fiction. The imagination involves abstract thought—it is abstract thought.

Damage to the frontal lobes results in an inability to think abstractly. In the years before brain imagery techniques, neurologists used a proverbs test to assess frontal lobe damage. If I ask you what this means, "Still waters run deep," you answer to the effect, "Quiet people are profound." And I ought to know. A person with frontal lobe damage answers in a concrete and literal manner, "When water doesn't move, it makes no noise." If I ask what this means, "Empty barrels make a lot of noise," you answer to the effect, "Dumb people talk a lot." And I wouldn't know anything about that. A person with frontal lobe damage answers, "An empty barrel makes more noise than a full barrel because there's no echo in a full barrel." This statement is correct, but it is not the meaning of the proverb.

I'll conclude by pointing out that everything we've done in this course involves abstract thought. I've been lecturing on topics none of which are physically present. You've been taking notes and thinking about things that are not physically present. This ability to think abstractly defines human beings in a fundamental manner. This characteristic is responsible for the success of our species. The ability to be in one place physically and to think of another place psychologically makes us who and what we are.

Thank you.

Tips to Students ~
Time Management

Successful performance in school is related to time management!

Never take more courses than you can handle. And never take a course at a time you know it will be difficult to attend.

Use travel time to your advantage. Study while waiting for buses and trains. Squeeze study time in whenever you have to wait or are delayed.

Get into the study habit. Block out slices of time on a daily basis that you can devote to study and to completing assignments. Future readings, tests, projects and assignments can be started long before the due date.

Read the syllabus for each course carefully. Know the dates for all tests and hand-in assignments. Never be caught unprepared.

Assess the amount of work you will need to complete to succeed on tests and on assignments. Long complex assignments can be broken down into shorter and simpler assignments mastered one step at a time. A term paper can be divided into smaller and manageable segments. A chapter of thirty pages can be read in one long tiring session or in five stress-free sessions of six pages a day.

Know the amount of time you can devote to course work on a daily basis. Be realistic in your estimates of work and time.

Buy a *day planner* and write down on a daily basis what you need to do. Try to do a little work everyday.

Organize assignments for all courses by date and then *prioritize*. Which assignments need to be completed first?

Putting assignments off to the last minute results in unnecessary stress and pressure. Putting assignments off often results in rushed and poorly prepared work that could have been improved.

There is no better time than the present to do class work. There is no time but the present. Don't believe that you can procrastinate and complete assignments by cramming at a later time.

Make sure you include in your daily planning time for fun, social events, exercise, and a sound night's sleep.

A Note on the Choice of the Cover Photograph

People who saw the cover photograph before the book was published remarked that it was bright and cheery and somewhat out of place in a dense intellectual tome. I suppose these people preferred a photograph of Rodin's *Thinker* or a photograph of the *Pensive Christ* that's carved in wood and sold in flea markets in Baltic old towns. I felt I needed to give an explanation for the choice of the photograph.

The photograph, which was taken some years ago in Oahu, provides the opportunity to speculate about the personality of the surfer. Who is he? What's his name? Where's he from? How old is he? What kind of person is he? Is he a friendly guy? Or is he unfriendly?—he's alone, after all. Can he surf? Or is he a poseur who strolls the beach board in hand, giving people the impression that he surfs when, in fact, he doesn't? Is he a tourist? Or is he a resident of Oahu? Did he go to college? If he did, what was his major? What does he do for a living? Does he have a job? Or is he a proverbial beach bum, living splendidly in the great outdoors? Does he have a girlfriend? Is he married? Does he have a family? Does he have siblings? Do they surf? Where do his parents live? What do his parents do for a living? We can go on with these questions all day long. If we were adherents of the psychodynamic perspective, we might supply answers to these questions through the accommodating process of projection.

The photograph allows us to progress from considering the particulars of an individual life to speculating about the psychological principles covered in Volume One. We can consider this solitary surfer in the light of the perspectives covered in Lecture One. Are there brain sites responsible for mastering the simmering gravity of a surfboard?

Does the proclivity to surf run in families? Did the ability to surf provide an evolutionary advantage to our ancestors? Is there a type of personality who seeks out the dangers and the thrills of surfing? What principles of learning underlie the behavior of surfing? What kind of mental discipline is required in surfing? Is there a culture of surfing and a surfing community of like-minded individuals?

We can consider the surfer in the light of the methods outlined in Lecture Two. Is there anything special about this surfer that would inspire a case study? What kind of surveys would we administer and correlate? To whom would we administer the surveys? What variables would we experiment on? The length of the board? The best stance on a board? The best way to capture a wave? The best training to compete in surfing contests?

We can consider the surfer through the principle of procedural long-term memory described in Lecture Three. This is memory for body movement and for locomotion. Procedural memory does not employ words—I suppose the only words spoken on a surfboard are "Yes!" for catching the big wave and "Oops!" for suffering a spill.

We can consider the surfer through the principles of learning described in Lecture Four. It must take years of practice to become a proficient surfer and it must take years of experience to discern the roll of the sea. Classical conditioning would have taught the surfer the once neutral signs of wind and sea and operant conditioning would have provided the reinforcement when he rode a wave to shore and the punishment when he didn't.

We can consider the surfer through the Big Five trait theory of personality reviewed in Lecture Five. He may be an introvert—he's alone on a beach. He has to be cooperative and agreeable with his fellow surfers. He may be open to experience new surfing techniques. He has to maintain a stable emotional state riding the surf, being neither too excitable nor too phlegmatic. And he has to be conscientious in trekking to the beach to master his technique.

Finally, we can consider the surfer through the neuroscience presented in Lecture Six. We can explore how the limbic system and the autonomic nervous system adjust as he emerges from a barrel of a maverick. And we can explore how the frontal lobes anticipate the dangers of the merciless ocean. Maybe that's why he's leaving a beach studded with a fat block of coral in the low tide.

From a single individual in a photograph we traverse a fertile ocean teeming with inquiries. There's another reason I chose this photograph for the cover. A 2008 study by Berman, Jonides and Kaplan entitled *Cognitive Benefit of Interacting with Nature* found that people who looked at photographs of nature while performing difficult intellectual chores exercised greater cognitive control in comparison to a control group that looked at photographs of crowded urban scenes.

Amid the strenuous mental task of contemplating these lectures, readers can fold the corner of the page, close the book, and daydream about surfing the North Shore of Oahu. Or, if you're like me, readers can daydream of watching someone surf the North Shore of Oahu. Our minds, if only temporarily, shift from dry intellectual pursuits to the possibility of hanging ten on a waxed deck in the warm white surf of Sunset Beach. Properly refreshed, we can reopen the book, fold back the page, and rejoin a voyage that has brought so many psychological marvels into our reckoning.